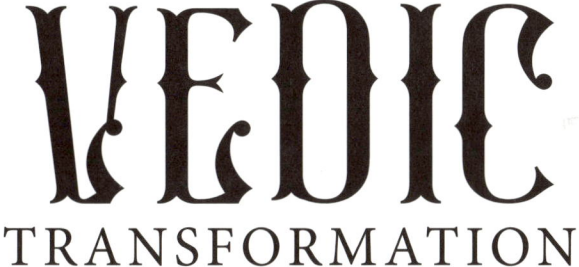

TRANSFORMATION

by

Vishnupriya Thacker

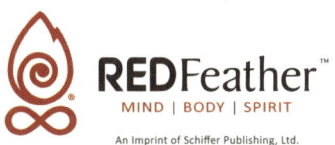

Copyright © 2022 by Vishnupriya Thacker

Library of Congress Control Number: 2021942581

All rights reserved. No part of this work may be reproduced or used in any form or by any means—graphic, electronic, or mechanical, including photocopying or information storage and retrieval systems—without written permission from the publisher.

The scanning, uploading, and distribution of this book or any part thereof via the Internet or any other means without the permission of the publisher is illegal and punishable by law. Please purchase only authorized editions and do not participate in or encourage the electronic piracy of copyrighted materials.

"Red Feather Mind Body Spirit" logo is a trademark of Schiffer Publishing, Ltd.
"Red Feather Mind Body Spirit Feather" logo is a registered trademark of Schiffer Publishing, Ltd.

Edited by James Young
Designed by Christopher Bower
Cover design by Brenda McCallum
Type set in Philosopher / Minion Pro

ISBN: 978-0-7643-6382-5
Printed in India

Published by REDFeather Mind, Body, Spirit
An imprint of Schiffer Publishing, Ltd.
4880 Lower Valley Road
Atglen, PA 19310
Phone: (610) 593-1777; Fax: (610) 593-2002
Email: Info@schifferbooks.com
Web: www.redfeathermbs.com

For our complete selection of fine books on this and related subjects, please visit our website at www.schifferbooks.com. You may also write for a free catalog.

Schiffer Publishing's titles are available at special discounts for bulk purchases for sales promotions or premiums. Special editions, including personalized covers, corporate imprints, and excerpts, can be created in large quantities for special needs. For more information, contact the publisher.

We are always looking for people to write books on new and related subjects. If you have an idea for a book, please contact us at proposals@schifferbooks.com.

Contents

Introduction 7

Chapter 1: The Correlation between Food and Emotions 8

Chapter 2: Gratitude 10

Chapter 3: Principles of Ayurveda 11

Chapter 4: Understanding Your Own *Prakruti*: Know Your Dosha 14

Chapter 5: Understanding the Importance of *Agni* 20

Chapter 6: Understanding the Importance of Water 22

Chapter 7: Food and the Six Tastes (*Rasa*) 24

Chapter 8: Ayurvedic Perspective on the
Consumption of Meat and Alcohol 27

Chapter 9: Food and Its Impact on Constitution 29

Chapter 10: Spices and Their Benefits 41

Chapter 11: Food Charts and Quantification 45

Chapter 12: Daily Intake Chart by Constitution 53

Chapter 13: Recipes 54

Chapter 14: Meal Plans by Dosha 89

Chapter 15: Moong Soup—Detox Therapy 92

Chapter 16: Panchakarma-Related Therapies 94

Chapter 17: Stress Reduction and Pranayama.............................96

Chapter 18: The Art of Mindfulness 101

Chapter 19: Understanding Chakra Energy 103

Chapter 20: Yoga Asanas to Improve *Agni* 106

Chapter 21: Common Ailments and the
Suggested Ayurvedic Remedies 107

Chapter 22: Understanding of Herbs...135

Chapter 23: Ayurvedic and Tantric View on Sexual Healing...................139

Chapter 24: Ongoing Maintenance as per Ayurveda.....................142

Conclusion 145

Notes 146

Glossary 147

Bibliography 154

Index..155

Acknowledgments

I am grateful to the Universe/Paramatma for the inspiration to create this guideline book. During the process, I was blessed with support from some incredible people and extend my heartfelt gratitude to my family and friends.

I would like to give a special note of appreciation to my close friend and respected Ayurvedacharya Dr. A. Bapat for her medical contribution, guidance, and expert Ayurvedic knowledge that helped me document certain nutritional concepts with a basic degree of scientific measurement.

I would like to clarify that I am an Ayurvedic wellness and spiritual healing coach (not an Ayurvedic doctor), and an avid practitioner of this age-old science, having benefited through my own personal experience by imbibing many of the principles illustrated in the following chapters. Thank you.

Namaste and love,

Vishnupriya.

Founder—Vedic Synergy, Inc.

https://www.vedicsynergy.com/

Introduction

Do you constantly feel exhausted and stressed?
Are you tired of counting calories every time you eat?
Do you feel that you lack a sense of total well-being?

The answers to the above questions can be found in this book, which has been designed as a practical reference guide to help you assimilate healthful living habits, taking into consideration your specific constitution, as outlined by the practice of Ayurveda—a five-thousand-year-old science from India. The chapters focus on concepts, suggestions, and techniques for increasing your well-being, not by counting calories but through sensual living and eating foods according to your specific constitution (*Dosha*). There are also home remedies and herbs suggested by an Ayurvedic doctor (*Ayurvedacharya*) for common ailments. In addition to nutritional guidelines, there are various spiritual healing concepts that have been described. All the concepts can be implemented easily and at your own pace for a complete mind-body-soul transformation.

The principles outlined in the following chapters are an essence of living, which has been left to us as a divine gift from the ancients. You will experience an inner well-being, filling your body and spirit with a renewed energy. On to chapter 1!

Each second you can be reborn. Each second there can be a new beginning. It is choice. It is your choice.[1]

—*Clearwater*

Namaste,
Vishnupriya

Chapter 1
The Correlation between Food and Emotions

Food affects us mentally, emotionally, and spiritually. The energies from nature are absorbed when natural foods are consumed, which affects a person's health and quality of life. In addition, the manner in which food is cooked, processed, and stored is crucial. For instance, if food is cooked patiently and with love, it will be more delicious.

Emotions rise spontaneously in response to situations in the past, in the present, or even in our imagination. Each feeling or emotion has its own energy quotient—and whatever we think, feel, consume, or even dream about will affect our well-being. There is a need to intuitively understand our feelings, since they influence our food choices.

If you are unaware of your emotions or feelings on a regular basis, there will be a subconscious need to suppress your pain, resulting in anxiety and undue stress. This in turn will make you lean toward foods that make you feel better, but could be unhealthful—such as sweets—on a regular basis. On the other hand, eating whole, natural, and light foods causes the mind to become calm, focused, and relaxed. If the food that is consumed is healthful, organic, and natural, food cravings for the "wrong foods" (processed foods or those that are not rejuvenating for your body) will diminish. According to Ayurveda, consuming foods in accordance with one's specific constitution brings about balance.

Ayurveda gives us further insight into the impact of foods on our thought processes and behaviors by delineating foods as *Sattvic, Rajasic, and Tamasic*. Sattvic foods tend to be natural, light, and healthy, fostering contentment, compassion, love, and forgiveness when consumed. Examples of Sattvic foods include green vegetables, whole grains, nuts, seeds, and fresh fruit. Rajasic foods are hot and spicy and tend to be salty. They are stimulants and can make an individual agitated or prone to anger, irritation, and manipulation. Onions and garlic are Rajasic foods. Tamasic foods tend to be heavy and induce sleep. They can cause stress and contribute to a less refined state of consciousness. Tamasic foods include red meat, fried food, and alcohol.

It is possible that at times, you may take a step backward and eat food items that are not healthful, as you did in the past; however, being present and persistent will make the transformation successful over time. The important point to remember is to always hear your own internal voice, evaluate how you feel after consuming a particular food item, and ensure that everything you put into your body—foods, emotions, and thoughts—is nourishing, in order to increase self-love. Your food choices will nourish you and affect the way you treat yourself and others on a moment-to-moment basis.

Chapter 2
Gratitude

Every morning a five-minute gratitude prayer allows one to feel grateful and happy for all the blessings that one has in their life. It brings about a sense of peace and reduces anxiety. Observe nature and become part of the environment, finding joy in the smallest of things—whether it is a child's laughter or seeing the changing colors of nature—and be grateful for being given the chance to enjoy another day in your life. This will help change your mood, reduce stress, put a smile on your face, and allow you to make more-healthful choices throughout the day.

Over time, gratitude leads to acts of kindness as simple as smiling and happily thanking the security guard at your office building for getting the elevator for you. This in turn will make him feel appreciated and grateful for his job. The act of extending appreciation to others helps us feel good from within and less anxious in general. Gratitude is a positive energy vibration that increases the more we embrace and practice it in our lives. It helps increase our self-confidence and diminishes the need to compare ourselves with others.

The result is that you will be more motivated to follow a more healthful lifestyle, work out, eat well, be more gentle and loving towards yourself. Instead of worrying about calories and strict diets, you will learn to see food in a way that satisfies all five senses. You will become more in tune with your own body's needs and learn to be grateful and appreciative of the taste, sight, smell, and feel of the food in your mouth. This will heighten the sense of satisfaction through the eyes, ears, mouth, nose, and hands, in keeping with the Ayurvedic concept of the five senses. Food is not to be eaten while on the run, but with a focus, in a quiet place, chewing each bite at least thirty-two times and savoring each mouthful with gratitude. If you start each meal with a gratitude prayer first, the food will be even more tasty. Try this out for yourself and experience the joy of savoring each delicious bite!

Chapter 3
Principles of Ayurveda

Ayurveda is an ancient science of life and medicine that originated in India more than five thousand years ago. The *Atharva Veda* describes over two hundred medicinal plants used by ancient Ayurvedic practitioners such as Charaka, Susruta, and Kasyapa. The most detailed text after the *Atharva Veda* was recorded by Charaka in the *Charaka Samhita*, which includes the principles derived from the Vedas, along with practical application. The practice was adopted by the Buddhists, who then spread the basic concepts to other countries such as Burma, Tibet, and Sri Lanka.

The word *Ayurveda* consists of *Ayu*, meaning the span of life, and *veda*, which means knowledge. It is the science of the *longevity of life*. The influence of Ayurveda as a healing science believes that mind, body, and spirit or consciousness need to be aligned and must be in harmony with all living beings and nature. This science provides us with a means to maintain optimum health and holistic well-being.

Life (Ayu) is the combination (Samyoga) of body, senses, mind, and reincarnating soul. Ayurveda is the most sacred science of life, beneficial to humans both in this world and the world beyond.[1]

—*Charaka Samhita, Sutrasthana, 1.42–43*

Ayurveda's holistic premise—that mind, body, and spirit are intimately connected—is revolutionizing our approach to health. Ayurveda teaches us that separating mind and spirit from the body creates physical imbalance, which is the first stage in the disease process; however, reintegration takes us toward complete healing, spiritual awareness, and bliss.

The goals of Ayurveda are the longevity and maintenance of a healthy life and prevention of disease, which allows one to focus on the four principal aims of life:
- ***Dharma***: virtue or duty
- ***Artha***: wealth
- ***Kama***: desire or love
- ***Moksha***: liberation or salvation

According to this science, everything in the Universe is composed of five elements: air, water, fire, earth, and space. These different elements combine to form the three *doshas—Vata, Pitta,* and *Kapha*—also known as the *metabolic types.* The doshas account for our individual differences and are based on bioindividuality rather than a "one size fits all" general concept. Any healing must take into account the physical, psychological, emotional, and spiritual well-being of a person according to Ayurveda, as well as the seasons and geographical locations, among other factors.

Ayurveda describes the entire physical universe, inclusive of human beings, in terms of the five elements or energetic patterns, also called *panchamahabhutas*—air, space, water, fire, and earth. Each cell in the human body is made up of these elements, which have specific functions to perform. The elements combine in various ways to form the metabolic types:
- *Vata:* air and space
- *Pitta:* fire and water
- *Kapha:* water and earth

The three doshas are present in all human beings in varying degrees, but there may be a dominance of one or two elements that make up our unique constitution or nature, known as *Prakruti*. An assessment of our most natural state would need to be undertaken to truly understand our dosha balance, or Prakruti.

In Ayurveda, ill health is considered as a dosha imbalance, or *Vikruti*. To treat this imbalance, Ayurveda aims to remove the root cause as the primary step in order to reestablish balance in the body.

Additionally, an imbalanced dosha can interrupt the natural flow of *Prana*, or vital life force or energy. The fundamental cause of any imbalance according to this ancient science is due to the imbalance in the person's digestive process, or digestive

Agni, which is responsible for the main functions of digestion and metabolism. If the digestive fire or Agni is weak, the body is overwhelmed by the buildup of internal toxins/waste, or *Ama*.

According to Ayurveda, the components of the body include the:
- three doshas (*Tridosha—Vata, Pitta, and Kapha*),
- seven tissues (*Saptadhatu*), and
- three waste products (*Malas*).

All three components need to be balanced in order to maintain a healthy body. It is focused on perfecting the body's biorhythm and metabolism—the breakdown and regrowth of cellular structures. Ayurvedic treatment by a qualified practitioner would include recommendations on nutrition, cleansing, herbs, yoga, meditation, and detox therapies (including massage).

Finally, the Ayurvedic philosophy believes that everything in the universe is interconnected and interrelated. We must live in accordance with the laws of nature and the cosmic rhythm to be happy and healthy. Health is when we are in balance internally as well as externally, and in harmony with the environment. It is when you are joyous, calm, and in a clear state of the body, mind, and spirit. Additionally, it is the balance of your constitution, bodily tissues, and your digestive process, resulting in increased energy, vitality, and radiance.

Chapter 4
Understanding your own *Prakruti*: Know Your Dosha

The source of all existence is universal cosmic consciousness, and it exists in all living organisms. Each macro and microorganism has a self-identity, containing the three universal qualities, or *Gunas*, contributing to the various aspects of perception:
- *Sattva*: creation
- *Rajas*: preservation
- *Tamas*: destruction or transformation

Ayurveda believes that everything in this universe, including each cell in the human body, is made up of five elements:
- **air:** oxygen is the basis for all energy movements.
- **space** or **ether:** in which everything happens and represents vibration.
- **fire:** has the power to transform the state of any substance in the body. Fire binds the atoms together and transforms food into energy.
- **water:** a large part of the body is made up of water. It represents the liquid state of substances such as blood.
- **earth:** is the solid state of matter in the body and provides stability, permanence, and rigidity.

As described in the previous chapter, the above five elements combine to form the three main doshas:

Vata: comprises *air and space* and is light, dry, cold, and rough. Vata regulates the principle of movement in the human body for functions such as chewing, swallowing, breathing, and peristalsis.

Vata Individual Characteristics:
Thin, delicate body structure, narrow limbs, dry hair and skin. The Vata-oriented individual has irregular digestion, eats frequently in small quantities, and is prone to constipation. Individuals with a dominant Vata dosha are analytical, innovative, creative, enthusiastic, and lively.

Pitta: comprises *fire and water* and is sharp, intense, and hot. Pitta regulates the transformation or conversion of substances in the human body including such functions as digestion, metabolism, temperature regulation, sensory perception, and understanding.

Pitta Individual Characteristics:
Medium build and weight; sharp with proportionate features; smooth, shiny skin and hair. A person with a dominant Pitta dosha has a sharp appetite, tends to feel hungry at short intervals, and digests food relatively quickly. A Pitta-oriented individual is focused, passionate, an initiator, leader, and a perfectionist, with a sharp, probing intellect. Pitta individuals may be prone to anger, competition, and jealousy.

Kapha: comprises *earth and water* and is heavy and slow. It relates to the structure, strength, and immunity of the body. Kapha body areas are the chest, lungs, and spinal fluid.

Kapha Individual Characteristics:
A large, plump frame with strong bones, thick hair and skin, and a slow metabolism makes them prone to gaining weight. Kapha individuals tend to avoid physical activity, making it harder for them to lose weight. People with a dominant Kapha dosha are warm, supportive, generous, and provide stability to family and friends, which allows them to form long-lasting relationships. They are excellent caregivers due to their calm and soothing personalities.

An assessment of Prakruti should take into consideration our physical structure, emotional makeup, and mental tendencies. The knowledge of one's Prakruti can aid in maintaining optimal health. In the following chart, please choose characteristics on the basis of your overall lifelong tendencies and not according to temporary or recent conditions.

Choose one from each row in each section. Count the number of characteristics you choose from each column in both sections. The column with highest score is indicative of your dominant constitution.

Physical Body:

Observation	Vata	Pitta	Kapha
Physique	Thin and lean—short or tall	Medium, toned, and proportionate	Heavy, plump, bulky, and broad
Voice	High pitch	Medium pitch	Low pitch
Hair volume	Thin	Average	Thick
Hair type	Dry	Normal	Oily
Skin type	Dry and rough	Normal	Oily
Body heat (skin)	Cold	Warm	Cool
Eyes	Small	Medium	Large
Whites of eyes	Brown tinge	Red tinge	Very white
Teeth	Small or very large	Medium	Large
Weight	Low body fat—does not put on easily	Medium—can gain over time	Heavy—puts on easily
Metabolism	Irregular	Strong	Slow
Sleep	Light and irregular	Sound	Heavy
Speech	Fast—can miss words	Sharp and precise	Sweet and slow
Elimination	Dry, hard, constipated	Soft and moist—multiple times during the day	Heavy and slow
Hunger and thirst	Irregular	Sharp—needs food when hungry and always thirsty	Can miss meals easily and steady thirst
Food and drink inclination	Warm/hot	Cold	Warm
Food—inclined toward	Creamy, sweet, spicy	Sweet and cold	Warm and spicy
Exercise tolerance	High	Medium	Low
Weather	Does not like the cold	Does not like heat	Does not like cool and damp

Understanding your own *Prakruti*: Know Your Dosha

Psychological body and personality:

Observation	Vata	Pitta	Kapha
Nature of dreams	Fearful	Angry and courageous/ daring	Loving and harmonious
Anger	Irregular	Quite often	Rarely
Patience	Irregular	Less	Strong
Personality	Nervous, fearful, creative	Intelligent, competitive, dynamic, arrogant, short temper	Calm, steady, greedy
Thoughts	Irregular and changing	Fairly steady	Steady and fixed
Confidence	Timid	Outwardly self-confident	Inwardly confident
Attainment of goals	Distracted	Focused	Steady
When intimidated	Run	Fight	Makes peace
Trauma causes	Anxiousness	Avoidance	Depression
Socially	Shy and lacking in confidence	Wants to be center of attention	Calm and relaxed
Spiritual	Inclined spiritually	Inclined to be materialistic and spiritual	Basically materialistic
Friendships	Makes friends easily	Friends connected to work, intense	Long-established friends
Affection expressed through	Words	Gifts	Touch
Personal relationship / partner	Clingy	Jealous	Secure
Prefers to work	Under supervision and direction	Alone	In groups
Competition	Dislikes	Driven	Handles well
Finances	Does not save	Saves and big spender	Saves regularly
Total			

Height-Weight Charts by Dosha

Understanding weight maintenance by height and by dosha is of crucial importance when undergoing a transformative process toward optimal health. The height-weight chart below is for *women* between the ages of *25–59 years*.[1]

Height	Small Frame (Weight in Pounds)	Dosha (Constitution)	Medium Frame (Weight in Pounds)	Dosha (Constitution)	Large Frame (Weight in Pounds)	Dosha (Constitution)
4'10"	102–111	Vata	109–121	Pitta	118–131	Kapha
4'11"	103–113	Vata	111–123	Pitta	120–134	Kapha
5'0"	104–115	Vata	113–126	Pitta	122–137	Kapha
5'1"	106–118	Vata	115–129	Pitta	125–140	Kapha
5'2"	108–121	Vata	118–132	Pitta	128–143	Kapha
5'3"	111–124	Vata	121–135	Pitta	131–147	Kapha
5'4"	114–127	Vata	124–138	Pitta	134–151	Kapha
5'5"	117–130	Vata	127–141	Pitta	137–155	Kapha
5'6"	120–133	Vata	130–144	Pitta	140–159	Kapha
5'7"	123–136	Vata	133–147	Pitta	143–163	Kapha
5'8"	126–139	Vata	136–150	Pitta	146–167	Kapha
5'9"	129–142	Vata	139–153	Pitta	149–170	Kapha
5'10"	132–145	Vata	142–156	Pitta	152–173	Kapha
5'11"	135–148	Vata	145–159	Pitta	155–176	Kapha
6'0"	138–151	Vata	148–162	Pitta	158–179	Kapha

Understanding your own *Prakruti*: Know Your Dosha

The height-weight chart below is for *men* between the ages of *25–59* years.[2]

Height	Small Frame (Weight in Pounds)	Dosha (Constitution)	Medium Frame (Weight in Pounds)	Dosha (Constitution)	Large Frame (Weight in Pounds)	Dosha (Constitution)
5'2"	128–134	Vata	131–141	Pitta	138–150	Kapha
5'3"	130–136	Vata	133–143	Pitta	140–153	Kapha
5'4"	132–138	Vata	135–145	Pitta	142–156	Kapha
5'5"	134–140	Vata	137–148	Pitta	144–160	Kapha
5'6"	136–142	Vata	139–151	Pitta	146–164	Kapha
5'7"	138–145	Vata	142–154	Pitta	149–168	Kapha
5'8"	140–148	Vata	145–157	Pitta	152–172	Kapha
5'9"	142–151	Vata	148–160	Pitta	155–176	Kapha
5'10"	144–154	Vata	151–163	Pitta	158–180	Kapha
5'11"	146–157	Vata	154–166	Pitta	161–184	Kapha
6'0"	149–160	Vata	157–170	Pitta	164–188	Kapha
6'1"	152–164	Vata	160–174	Pitta	168–192	Kapha
6'2"	155–168	Vata	164–178	Pitta	172–197	Kapha
6'3"	158–172	Vata	167–182	Pitta	176–202	Kapha
6'4"	162–176	Vata	171–187	Pitta	181–207	Kapha

Chapter 5
Understanding the Importance of *Agni*

Agni (fire) is responsible for transmutation and is considered to be one of the governing principles in the body. The main function of Agni is to digest and transform food into *Ojas*, or energy/immunity. Ayurveda focuses on the quality of Agni in the body, the primary responsibility of which is the digestion and transformation of matter into energy, cellular growth, and sensations into consciousness.

If the Agni is in good condition in the body, then there is a balance in the doshas, tissues, and *Malas*, or waste products. The person has strong immunity and is considered healthy. It is possible for each of us during this transformative journey to reach this state of optimum health, both internally and externally. Ayurveda's three main principles—maintenance, prevention, and healing—are based on the strength and quality of fire in the body. Agni is also considered to be the biological conduit that connects the mind and body to the Universe.

According to Ayurveda, most disorders in the body are due to the imbalance of Agni. Undigested food, thoughts, and emotions accumulate to form *Ama*, or toxins, and this in turn generates gas, bloating, fatigue, rashes, pains, etc., which are the indicators of an unhealthy body. The fermentation of undigested or semi-digested food gives rise to hyperacidity in the gastrointestinal tract. In addition, Ama also circulates in the body and gets attached to the weakest organs, resulting in imbalances such as kidney stones, cellulite, and rheumatoid arthritis.

An imbalanced fire is evident in the body's aura, intelligence, beauty, and shine. It can cause fear, anxiousness, laziness, and impatience, which restrict a person's ability to deal with life situations. The results are a lack of clarity, compassion, and love, both professionally and personally. Such imbalances in the fire can be rectified by modification in diet, exercise, meditation, and *Pranayama* (breathing techniques) as per the individual's constitution. If this is not sufficient, then a detox, or *Panchakarma*, is advised. During this process, the toxins are removed from the body, followed by rejuvenation (*rasayana*) therapy to tone up the muscles and strengthen Agni.

Individuals with a Vata constitution have an erratic Agni—there is variable digestion, and the metabolic function can slow down. *Vishamagni*, or irregular digestion, in Vata individuals can cause constipation, colic pain, gurgling sounds in the intestine, gas, lower backache, and insomnia. Emotionally, it can make one fearful or anxious.

Individuals with a Pitta constitution have a sharp and fiery (*Tiksha*) Agni. In this instance, the fire becomes intense and causes hypermetabolism, stimulating more enzyme secretion. This causes a burning sensation in the chest and stomach, as well as acid reflux, and increases thirst. Hunger pangs are usually sharp and often accompanied by a headache. Emotionally, it can make one angry, envious, and judgmental.

Individuals with a Kapha constitution have a slow (*Manda*) Agni, resulting in a prolonged digestive process. This can cause nausea, excess saliva, laziness, and a sense of heaviness in the stomach. Emotionally, one can become needy and possessive.

A balanced Agni is when food is digested well to produce *Ojas* (immunity), *Tejas* (metabolic strength), and *Prana* (life force). The importance of the quality of fire in the body cannot be overemphasized, since it is responsible for a number of bodily functions, including:

- digestion and assimilation of food, resulting in the nutrition of the body and visual perception.
- the body temperature, color, complexion, and clarity of the skin.
- *Tejas*, which is a requirement for all cellular metabolic activity, including reasoning capacity of the mind and discrimination.
- the lifespan of the body, including vitality, strength, confidence, and a healthy glow.

Once the Agni is at its optimum state for the body, you will feel healthy, radiant, energetic, and happy.

Chapter 6
Understanding the Importance of Water

Our bodies consist of 75 percent water. It is a commonly known fact that drinking more water will help us lose weight. Every nutritional or weight-loss program emphasizes drinking about eight glasses of water daily.

Let's understand why drinking water is so important for the body. Water is known to be an appetite suppressant and helps the body metabolize stored fat. It is important to drink enough water to have normal bowel movements in order to avoid constipation (especially during the cold season), gas, bloating, and dry skin. Water intake moisturizes skin from within and makes it glow.

Water is needed for the kidneys to function efficiently and to assist in the removal of toxins from the body. If you drink more water, this will allow the retained water (water weight) to be released from the body. This in turn prevents dehydration and protects the liver. Dehydration slows down the fat-burning process, reduces the amount of oxygen reaching the muscles, and causes fatigue. When you drink the recommended amount of water, you are aiding the process of blood circulation, maintaining the right body temperature, and lowering the possibility of joint soreness while exercising. One of the biggest benefits of drinking water is that it has a positive impact on your attitude, emotions, and overall well-being.

It is suggested to calculate the amount of water intake on the basis of body weight, activity levels, activity intensity, temperature, humidity of the environment, and diet. It is imperative to understand that caffeinated drinks (coffee, tea, soda) and alcohol cause the body to flush out water. To compensate for the effect of these diuretics, it is suggested to consume more water.

Many people misinterpret low energy levels as hunger for food rather than realizing that dehydration is setting in, and all the body needs is more water. Several studies have been done where individuals were advised to have water at the first sign of hunger instead of eating food, resulting in more weight loss. The suggestion in Ayurveda is to drink room-temperature water fifteen minutes prior to a meal.

Ayurveda has given us some specific recommendations regarding the intake of water:

- Ayurveda encourages the individual to identify the subtle signals provided by one's body, and to drink water whenever thirsty. Thirst has become one of the more commonly suppressed natural urges, so listening to the body's need for hydration is important. Pitta (due to the fire element) and Vata (due to the dry air element) individuals need to drink more water to keep the body hydrated.
- Ayurveda advises that having a glass of warm or room-temperature water first thing in the morning upon waking up is beneficial for health. This stimulates the gastrointestinal tract and the peristalsis motion (muscle contractions within the intestinal walls).
- This science does not recommend cold water or any iced drinks or sodas. In fact, it suggests drinking warm or room-temperature water to balance all three doshas, cleanse the gastrointestinal tract, enhance digestion, boost the metabolic rate, and improve immunity.

Chapter 7
Food and the Six Tastes (*Rasa*)

Ayurveda puts emphasis on understanding our doshas and the principle of taste, or *Rasa*. Rasa means essence. Rasa has a direct correlation to one's dosha, since the consumption of certain foods with a specific Rasa can increase or decrease the essential elements of the dosha, causing an imbalance. The tastes that share a common element with the dosha aggravate it, and those with contrasting elements decrease it. To elucidate, an increased consumption of foods with a sweet taste by an individual with the Kapha constitution, for example, will actually increase the Kapha characteristics in the body, resulting in weight gain. In accordance with Ayurveda, a balanced intake of each of the six rasas will result in the proper functioning of the different organs of the body.

It begins with the taste in the tongue, one of the five senses. However, as it flows through the digestive process, Rasa has either a heating or cooling effect on the body. The energy that is felt immediately after eating a food item is known as *Virya*. Every taste also has a long-term effect on our metabolism after the digestive process is completed and the nutrients have been absorbed, known as *Vipaka*.

The six rasas in Ayurveda are:
- *Amla* or sour
- *Madhura* or sweet
- *Lavana* or salty
- *Tikta* or bitter
- *Katu* or pungent
- *Kasaya* or astringent

It is essential to understand the effects of each of the six tastes on the body. The sweet taste, for example, satisfies the senses, calms the nerves, and emotionally increases the sense of security and love in an individual. The pungent taste reduces fat in the body and cures respiratory infection. Emotionally, the pungent taste is known to increase clarity, focus, excitement, and stubbornness.

Let's understand the impact of each of these tastes on the doshas and the foods that constitute the different tastes:

Taste	Food Source	Effect on Dosha—Increases	Effect on Dosha—Decreases
Sweet	Milk, sweet fruit, and root vegetables	Kapha	Pitta and Vata
Sour	Citrus fruits, green grapes, and pickles	Pitta and Kapha	Vata
Salty	Natural salts, sea vegetables, and cheese	Pitta and Kapha	Vata
Bitter	Dark leafy vegetables, spices, vegetables such as bitter gourd, and grapefruit	Vata	Pitta and Kapha
Pungent	Garlic, chili peppers, ginger, raw onions, radishes, and mustard greens	Pitta and Vata	Kapha
Astringent	Legumes, walnuts, cashews, green bananas, okra, and alfalfa sprouts	Vata	Pitta and Kapha

Diet with the six tastes is satisfying and brings about a balance in our actions, moods, and lifestyle. Imbalances in the three doshas can be pacified by the different tastes as follows:

- *Pitta:* can be pacified by having foods with sweet, bitter, and astringent tastes.
- *Vata:* can be pacified by having foods with sweet, sour, and salty tastes.
- *Kapha:* can be pacified by having foods with pungent, bitter, and astringent tastes.

Tastes have an impact on weight management. Foods can be categorized by the speed at which they are absorbed by the blood stream after eating, better known as the *glycemic index*. Foods that enter the blood stream quickly have a higher glycemic index. The greater the insulin response, the more weight you can gain. The tastes that increase our weight are sweet, salty, and sour.

Eating habits that affect weight in the body can be separated into two kinds:

- The first is *head hunger*, where in order to deal with emotions such as anger, stress, frustration, bitterness, and resentment you may tend to lean toward foods with sour and pungent tastes. To deal with head hunger, it is advised to try to move away from the thoughts of food and focus on Pranayama and meditation practices instead, which will allow you to center yourself to become calm.
- With the second kind, *heart hunger*, you may choose foods with sweet and astringent tastes. Emotional needs cause cravings that can be tackled by resorting to positive diversions such as listening to music or speaking with a friend, rather than sweet foods. This will distract you from reaching for desserts, and when you are emotionally calmer, you may either not need to eat anything or may choose a healthful snack such as fruit instead.

Chapter 8
Ayurvedic Perspective on the Consumption of Meat and Alcohol

In Ayurveda, the gastrointestinal tract and digestion are the basis for good health. Simply put, heavy foods are more difficult to digest than lighter foods. The heaviness of meat dulls the digestion, reducing the speed and alertness of one's mental faculties. An imbalanced digestive fire (*Agni*) weakens the digestive process and creates toxins in the body, resulting in lethargy, increased thirst, and heartburn.

Food has three qualities (*Gunas*) as per the ancient science of Ayurveda—*Sattvic*, *Rajasic*, and *Tamasic*. Meat and alcohol fall into the category of Tamasic foods, since they do not induce positive, noble thoughts when ingested. In fact, when consumed they increase the negative emotions of anger and aggression. This becomes even more critical if the consumed meat is not organic, since the animal has likely been injected with steroids. It is also important to consider how the animal is slaughtered, since stress hormones are released at that time, affecting the quality of the meat. We absorb the intrinsic quality (*guna*) of the food that we eat, which, in turn, affects our behavior.

The ancient texts do not indicate that the eating of meat was banned in ancient times, but it was advised that it should be eaten only as a medicine or given only to those engaged in excessive physical activity (e.g., warriors in that time period) or to those who tend to overexert themselves. If meat is consumed without enough physical exercise, it can slow down the metabolic rate and increase toxins (*Ama*) and fat in the body. Therefore, vegetarian food is considered to be pure (*Sattvic*) in nature and is encouraged. If one is unable to eliminate meat from the diet, the suggestion is to reduce the intake. As an example, it might be good to try eating one vegetarian meal and the other as a chicken soup or broth to slowly get into the practice of reducing the intake of meat. Red meat should be avoided, and if meat is consumed, it is suggested to be eaten at the right time (during the day—avoid in the evenings) and in limited quantity.

In Ayurveda, alcohol is considered to be a toxin. The qualities of alcohol are the opposite of Ojas (immunity)—when consumed it causes agitation, adds fire in the body, and can lead to negative emotions. Excessive intake of alcohol is cautioned against, since it has the ability to reach the heart quickly and directly. It was the practice to consume alcohol only as a medicine—it was made from sugar, fruits, and grains and often was mixed with herbs for their healing effects. In the ancient texts, alcohol is not considered to be Sattvic, since it has the ability to affect your peace of mind and hamper the attainment of spiritual enlightenment.

In our modern world, we are becoming cognizant of the fact that a higher state of consciousness has a positive, healing benefit on the mind, body, and soul, bringing about balance and harmony. The ancient science of Ayurveda had already understood this fundamental concept—that enhancing the spiritual and higher consciousness in a human being would in turn bring about balance in the body, resulting in overall wellness.

Chapter 9
Food and Its Impact on Constitution

The table below provides details for the different natural food items by category—their taste (Rasa) and their impact on the three doshas (Vata, Pitta, Kapha). To illustrate by an example, consuming horseradish would help in balancing Kapha (comprising the earth and water elements), since foods that have bitter (air and space elements), pungent (fire and air elements), and astringent (air and earth elements) tastes are good for reducing Kapha. [Note: It is possible that the initial taste of a food item that is raw may change once cooked.]

Name of Food	Predominant Rasa	Impact on Constitution
Root Vegetables:		
Beetroot	Sweet, bitter	Increases Kapha; decreases Vata, Pitta
Burdock root	Astringent, bitter, sweet	Increases Vata; decreases Pitta, Kapha
Carrot (raw)	Sweet, bitter, pungent	Increases Kapha; decreases Vata, Pitta
Horseradish	Bitter, pungent	Increases Vata, Pitta; decreases Kapha
Jicama	Astringent, sweet	Increases Kapha; decreases Vata, Pitta
Onions	Pungent, sweet	Increases Vata, Pitta; decreases Kapha
Parsnip	Bitter, pungent, sweet	Increases Vata, Pitta; decreases Kapha
Potato (white)	Astringent, sweet	Increases Vata; decreases Pitta, Kapha
Radish	Pungent, bitter	Increases Vata, Pitta; decreases Kapha
Sweet potato	Sweet	Increases Kapha; decreases Vata, Pitta
Turnip	Astringent, pungent	Increases Vata, Pitta; decreases Kapha
Yam	Sweet	Increases Kapha; decreases Vata, Pitta

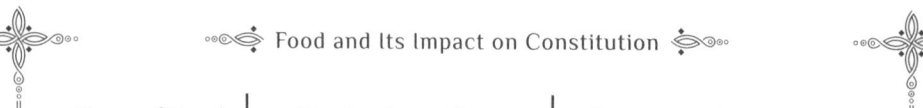
Food and Its Impact on Constitution

Name of Food	Predominant Rasa	Impact on Constitution
Stem Vegetables:		
Asparagus	Astringent, sweet	Increases Vata; decreases Pitta, Kapha
Celery stalk	Bitter, pungent	Increases Vata, Pitta; decreases Kapha
Leeks (raw)	Pungent, sweet	Increases Kapha; decreases Vata, Pitta
Rhubarb	Astringent, bitter, pungent	Decreases Vata, Pitta, Kapha
Scallion	Bitter, pungent, sweet	Increases Pitta; decreases Vata, Kapha
Leafy Vegetables:		
Alfalfa sprouts	Astringent, bitter	Increases Vata; decreases Pitta, Kapha
Arugula	Bitter	Increases Vata; decreases Pitta, Kapha
Basil	Sweet, pungent, bitter	Increases Pitta; decreases Vata, Kapha
Collard greens	Astringent, bitter	Increases Vata; decreases Pitta, Kapha
Dandelion greens	Bitter, pungent	Increases Vata; decreases Pitta, Kapha
Grape leaves	Astringent	Increases Vata; decreases Pitta, Kapha
Kale	Bitter	Increases Vata; decreases Pitta, Kapha
Lettuce	Astringent, bitter	Increases Vata; decreases Pitta, Kapha
Mustard leaves	Bitter, pungent	Increases Vata, Pitta; decreases Kapha
Spinach	Astringent, bitter, pungent, sweet	Increases Vata, Kapha; decreases Pitta
Swiss chard	Bitter	Increases Vata; decreases Pitta, Kapha
Watercress	Astringent, bitter	Increases Vata, Pitta; decreases Kapha

Food and Its Impact on Constitution

Name of Food	Predominant Rasa	Impact on Constitution
Flower Vegetables:		
Artichokes	Astringent, bitter	Increases Vata; decreases Pitta, Kapha
Broccoli	Bitter, sweet	Increases Vata; decreases Pitta, Kapha
Brussel sprouts	Astringent, bitter	Increases Vata, Pitta; decreases Kapha
Cabbage	Astringent, pungent, sweet	Increases Vata; decreases Pitta, Kapha
Cauliflower	Astringent, sweet	Increases Vata; decreases Pitta, Kapha
Fruit Vegetables:		
Avocado	Sweet	Increases Kapha; decreases Vata, Pitta
Bell pepper	Bitter, pungent, sweet	Increases Vata, Pitta; decreases Kapha
Bitter gourd/melon	Bitter	Increases Vata; decreases Pitta, Kapha
Bottle gourd	Sweet	Increases Kapha; decreases Vata, Pitta
Cucumber	Astringent, bitter, sweet	Increases Vata, Kapha; decreases Pitta
Eggplant	Bitter, pungent, sweet	Increases Vata, Pitta; decreases Kapha
Pumpkin	Sweet	Increases Kapha; decreases Vata, Pitta
Olives	Bitter, salty, sour	Increases Pitta, Kapha; decreases Vata
Squash (summer)	Sweet	Increases Kapha; decreases Vata, Pitta
Corn (sweet)	Sweet	Increases Vata, Kapha; decreases Pitta
Tomato (raw)	Pungent, sour, sweet	Increases Vata, Pitta; decreases Kapha
Zucchini	Astringent, sweet	Decreases Vata, Pitta, Kapha

Food and Its Impact on Constitution

Name of Food	Predominant Rasa	Impact on Constitution
Podded Vegetables:		
Drumstick	Astringent, bitter, pungent	Increases Pitta; decreases Vata, Kapha
Green beans	Astringent, bitter	Decreases Vata, Pitta, Kapha
Sweet peas	Sweet	Increases Vata, Kapha; decreases Pitta
Okra (cooked)	Astringent, sweet	Decreases Vata, Pitta, Kapha
Fruits:		
Apple (raw)	Astringent, sour, sweet	Increases Vata; decreases Pitta, Kapha
Apricot	Astringent, sour, sweet	Increases Pitta; decreases Vata, Kapha
Banana	Sweet, sour	Increases Kapha; decreases Vata, Pitta
Blackberry	Astringent, sour, sweet	Increases Kapha; decreases Vata, Pitta
Blueberries	Astringent, sour, sweet	Increases Kapha; decreases Vata, Pitta
Cantaloupe	Sweet	Increases Kapha; decreases Vata, Pitta
Cherries	Sour, sweet	Increases Pitta; decreases Vata, Kapha
Coconut	Sweet	Increases Kapha; decreases Vata, Pitta
Cranberries	Astringent, sour	Increases Vata; decreases Pitta, Kapha
Custard apple	Sweet	Increases Kapha; decreases Vata, Pitta
Date (dried)	Sweet	Increases Vata, Kapha; decreases Pitta
Fig (fresh)	Sweet, astringent	Increases Kapha; decreases Vata, Pitta
Gooseberry	Sour	Decreases Vata, Pitta, Kapha
Grapes	Sour, sweet	Increases Kapha; decreases Vata, Pitta
Grapefruit	Bitter, sour, sweet	Increases Pitta; decreases Vata, Kapha

Food and Its Impact on Constitution

Name of Food	Predominant Rasa	Impact on Constitution
\multicolumn{3}{c}{*Fruits: (Continued)*}		
Kiwi	Sour, sweet	Increases Pitta, Kapha; decreases Vata
Lemon	Astringent, bitter, salty, sour	Increases Pitta; decreases Vata, Kapha (in moderation)
Lime	Bitter, sweet	Decreases Vata, Pitta, Kapha (in moderation)
Lychee	Sweet	Increases Kapha; decreases Vata, Pitta
Mango (ripe)	Sweet	Increases Pitta, Kapha; decreases Vata
Watermelon	Sweet	Increases Vata; decreases Pitta, Kapha
Mulberries	Astringent, sour, sweet	Increases Kapha; decreases Vata, Pitta
Honeydew melon	Sour, sweet	Increases Kapha; decreases Vata, Pitta
Orange	Sour, sweet	Increases Pitta; decreases Vata, Kapha
Papaya	Bitter, pungent, sweet	Increases Pitta, Kapha; decreases Vata
Peach	Astringent, sour, sweet	Increases Pitta, Kapha; decreases Vata
Pear	Astringent, sweet	Increases Vata; decreases Pitta, Kapha
Pineapple	Pungent, sour, sweet	Increases Pitta, Kapha; decreases Vata
Plum	Astringent, sour, sweet	Increases Pitta, Kapha; decreases Vata
Pomegranate	Astringent, sour, sweet	Decreases Vata, Pitta, Kapha
Prune (dried)	Sweet	Increases Vata; decreases Pitta, Kapha
Raspberry	Astringent, sour, sweet	Increases Pitta; decreases Vata, Kapha
Strawberry	Sweet, sour, astringent	Increases Pitta; decreases Vata, Kapha
Sugarcane	Sweet	Increases Kapha; decreases Vata, Pitta
Water chestnuts	Astringent, sweet	Increases Vata, Kapha; decreases Pitta

Food and Its Impact on Constitution

Name of Food	Predominant Rasa	Impact on Constitution
Nuts:		
Almonds (with skin)	Sweet, astringent, bitter	Increases Kapha; decreases Vata, Pitta
Brazil nuts	Sweet, astringent, bitter	Increases Vata, Kapha; decreases Pitta
Cashews	Sweet	Increases Pitta, Kapha; decreases Vata
Hazelnuts	Sweet, astringent, bitter	Increases Pitta, Kapha; decreases Vata
Macadamia nuts	Sweet, astringent, bitter	Increases Vata, Kapha; decreases Pitta
Peanuts	Astringent, sweet	Increases Vata, Pitta, Kapha
Pecans	Sweet, astringent, bitter	Increases Vata, Pitta; decreases Kapha
Pistachios	Bitter, sweet	Increases Vata, Pitta, Kapha
Pine nuts	Sweet, astringent	Increases Pitta, Kapha; decreases Vata
Walnuts	Sweet, astringent, bitter	Increases Vata, Pitta; decreases Kapha
Seeds:		
Chia seeds	Sweet	Increases Kapha; decreases Vata, Pitta
Hemp seeds	Sweet	Increases Kapha; decreases Vata, Pitta
Flaxseed	Sweet	Increases Kapha; decreases Vata, Pitta
Pumpkin seeds	Bitter, sweet	Decreases Vata, Pitta, Kapha
Poppy seeds	Astringent, sweet	Increases Kapha; decreases Vata, Pitta
Sesame seeds	Astringent, bitter, pungent, sweet	Increases Pitta, Kapha; decreases Vata
Sunflower seeds	Bitter, pungent, sweet	Increases Pitta, Kapha; decreases Vata

Food and Its Impact on Constitution

Name of Food	Predominant Rasa	Impact on Constitution
Grains:		
Amaranth	Astringent, sweet	Increases Vata; decreases Pitta, Kapha
Barley	Astringent, pungent, sweet	Increases Vata; decreases Pitta, Kapha
Brown rice	Sweet	Increases Pitta; decreases Vata, Kapha
Buckwheat	Astringent, pungent, sweet	Increases Vata, Pitta; decreases Kapha
Cream of wheat	Sweet	Increases Kapha; decreases Vata, Pitta
Kamut	Sweet	Increases Kapha; decreases Vata, Pitta
Millet	Astringent, sweet	Increases Vata, Pitta; decreases Kapha
Oats/oatmeal	Sweet	Increases Kapha; decreases Vata, Pitta
Quinoa	Bitter, sweet	Decreases Vata, Pitta, Kapha
Rice (basmati)	Astringent, sweet	Increases Kapha; decreases Vata, Pitta
Rye	Astringent, sweet	Increases Vata, Pitta; decreases Kapha
Spelt	Astringent, pungent, sweet	Increases Kapha; decreases Vata, Pitta
Tapioca	Sweet	Increases Kapha; decreases Vata, Pitta
Teff	Astringent, pungent	Increases Vata, Pitta; decreases Kapha
Wheat bran	Sweet	Increases Kapha; decreases Vata, Pitta
Whole wheat flour	Sweet	Increases Kapha; decreases Vata, Pitta

Food and Its Impact on Constitution

Name of Food	Predominant Rasa	Impact on Constitution
Dairy:		
Almond milk	Sweet	Increases Kapha; decreases Vata, Pitta
Buffalo's milk	Sweet	Increases Kapha; decreases Vata, Pitta
Butter (unsalted)	Sweet	Increases Kapha; decreases Vata, Pitta
Buttermilk	Sour, astringent	Increases Pitta, Kapha; decreases Vata
Cheese (soft)	Sour, salty	Increases Pitta, Kapha; decreases Vata
Cottage cheese	Sour	Increases Pitta, Kapha; decreases Vata
Cow's milk	Sweet	Increases Kapha; decreases Vata, Pitta
Egg whites	Sweet, astringent	Increases Vata, Kapha; decreases Pitta
Egg yolk	Salty, sweet	Increases Pitta, Kapha; decreases Vata
Frozen yogurt	Sweet	Increases Kapha; decreases Vata, Pitta
Ghee	Sweet	Increases Kapha (in excess); decreases Vata, Pitta
Goat's milk	Astringent, sweet	Increases Vata; decreases Pitta, Kapha
Ice cream	Sweet	Increases Kapha; decreases Vata (in moderation), Pitta
Rice milk	Sweet	Increases Kapha; decreases Vata, Pitta
Skim milk	Sweet	Increases Kapha; decreases Vata, Pitta
Soy cheese	Astringent, sour	Increases Pitta, Kapha; decreases Vata
Sour cream	Sour	Increases Pitta, Kapha; decreases Vata (in moderation)
Tofu	Astringent, sweet	Increases Vata, Kapha; decreases Pitta
Heavy (whipping) **cream**	Sweet	Increases Kapha; decreases Vata, Pitta
Yogurt/curd	Sour	Increases Pitta, Kapha; decreases Vata

Name of Food	Predominant Rasa	Impact on Constitution
Sweeteners:		
Barley malt syrup	Sweet	Increases Kapha; decreases Vata, Pitta
Brown sugar	Sweet	Increases Kapha; decreases Vata, Pitta
Date sugar	Sweet	Increases Kapha; decreases Vata, Pitta
Honey	Astringent, sweet	Increases Vata, Pitta; decreases Kapha
Jaggery/gur	Bitter, sour, sweet	Increases Pitta, Kapha; decreases Vata
Maple syrup	Sweet	Increases Kapha; decreases Vata, Pitta
White sugar	Sweet	Increases Kapha; decreases Vata, Pitta
Beans and Legumes:		
Adzuki beans	Astringent, pungent	Increases Vata, Kapha; decreases Pitta
Black beans	Astringent	Increases Vata; decreases Pitta, Kapha
Black-eyed peas	Astringent, sweet	Increases Vata; decreases Pitta, Kapha
Cannellini beans	Astringent	Increases Vata; decreases Pitta, Kapha
Chickpeas	Astringent	Increases Vata, Kapha; decreases Pitta
Fava beans	Astringent	Increases Vata, Kapha; decreases Pitta
Kidney beans	Astringent	Increases Vata, Kapha; decreases Pitta
Red lentils (masoor)	Astringent, sweet	Increases Vata; decreases Pitta, Kapha
Lima beans	Astringent	Increases Vata; decreases Pitta, Kapha
Mung beans	Astringent, sweet	Increases Vata; decreases Pitta, Kapha
Navy beans	Astringent	Increases Vata; decreases Pitta, Kapha
Pinto beans	Astringent	Increases Vata; decreases Pitta, Kapha
Soybeans	Astringent	Increases Vata; decreases Pitta, Kapha
Urad dal	Astringent, sweet	Increases Pitta, Kapha; decreases Vata
White kidney beans	Astringent	Increases Vata, Kapha; decreases Pitta
Yellow lentils (toor)	Astringent	Increases Vata; decreases Pitta, Kapha

Food and Its Impact on Constitution

Name of Food	Predominant Rasa	Impact on Constitution
Nonvegetarian:		
Beef	Sweet	Increases Pitta, Kapha; decreases Vata
Chicken	Sweet	Increases Pitta, Kapha; decreases Vata
Duck	Sweet	Increases Pitta, Kapha; decreases Vata
Fish (freshwater)	Sweet	Increases Kapha; decreases Vata, Pitta
Lamb	Sweet	Increases Pitta, Kapha; decreases Vata
Pork	Salty, sweet	Increases Pitta, Kapha; decreases Vata
Rabbit	Sweet	Increases Vata, Pitta; decreases Kapha
Turkey	Sweet	Increases Vata, Pitta; decreases Kapha
Oils:		
Almond oil	Sweet	Increases Kapha; decreases Vata, Pitta
Corn oil	Astringent, sweet	Increases Vata, Pitta, Kapha
Coconut oil	Sweet	Increases Kapha; decreases Vata, Pitta
Mustard oil	Pungent	Increases Pitta; decreases Vata, Kapha
Olive oil	Bitter, pungent	Increases Pitta, Kapha; decreases Vata
Peanut oil	Pungent, sweet	Increases Pitta; decreases Vata, Kapha
Safflower oil	Astringent, sweet	Increases Pitta, Kapha; decreases Vata
Sesame oil	Astringent, bitter, sweet	Increases Pitta; decreases Vata, Kapha
Sunflower oil	Astringent, sweet	Increases Kapha; decreases Vata, Pitta

Food and Its Impact on Constitution

Name of Food	Predominant Rasa	Impact on Constitution
Spices:		
Ajwain / carom seed	Bitter, pungent	Increases Pitta; decreases Vata, Kapha
Asafoetida	Bitter, pungent	Increases Pitta; decreases Vata, Kapha
Basil (fresh)	Bitter, pungent, sweet	Increases Pitta; decreases Vata, Kapha
Bay leaves	Pungent, sweet	Increases Pitta; decreases Vata, Kapha
Black pepper	Pungent	Increases Pitta; decreases Vata, Kapha
Black salt	Pungent, salty	Increases Pitta, Kapha; decreases Vata
Cardamom	Sweet, bitter, pungent, astringent	Decreases Vata, Pitta, Kapha
Cinnamon	Bitter, pungent, sweet	Increases Pitta; decreases Vata, Kapha
Cloves	Astringent, pungent	Increases Pitta (in excess); decreases Vata, Kapha
Coriander	Astringent, sweet	Increases Vata; decreases Pitta, Kapha
Cumin	Bitter, pungent	Increases Pitta; decreases Vata, Kapha
Curry leaves	Astringent, bitter, pungent	Increases Pitta; decreases Vata, Kapha
Dill	Bitter, pungent	Increases Pitta; decreases Vata, Kapha
Fennel seeds	Sweet, bitter, astringent	Decreases Vata, Pitta, Kapha
Fenugreek	Bitter, pungent, sweet	Increases Pitta; decreases Vata, Kapha

Food and Its Impact on Constitution

Name of Food	Predominant Rasa	Impact on Constitution
Spices: (Continued)		
Garlic	Astringent, bitter, pungent, sweet	Increases Pitta; decreases Vata, Kapha
Ginger (fresh)	Pungent	Increases Pitta; decreases Vata, Kapha
Green chilies	Pungent	Increases Pitta; decreases Vata, Kapha
Kokum (unripe)	Astringent, pungent, sour, sweet	Increases Kapha; decreases Vata, Pitta
Mint	Pungent, sweet	Increases Vata (in excess); decreases Pitta, Kapha
Mustard seeds (brown)	Bitter, pungent	Increases Pitta; decreases Vata, Kapha
Nutmeg	Astringent, bitter, pungent	Increases Pitta, Kapha; decreases Vata
Red chili powder	Pungent	Increases Pitta; decreases Vata, Kapha
Rosemary	Bitter, pungent	Increases Pitta; decreases Vata, Kapha
Saffron	Astringent, bitter, sweet	Increases Pitta; decreases Vata, Kapha
Tamarind	Sour, sweet	Increases Pitta, Kapha; decreases Vata
Thyme	Pungent	Increases Pitta; decreases Vata, Kapha
Turmeric	Astringent, bitter, pungent	Increases Pitta; decreases Vata, Kapha

Note: Milk should not be consumed with sour, bitter, salty, astringent, and pungent tastes, so combining milk with a meal is not advised.

Chapter 10
Spices and Their Benefits

The spice box, also called the *masala dabba*, is an integral part of the Indian kitchen. Spices are best stored in airtight containers. The different colors, varieties, and textures enhance the taste of the food being prepared but are also beneficial for our health. The spices have been part of the Indian cultural diaspora for more than five thousand years, as long as Ayurveda has been followed as a natural healing practice.

The list below highlights the seventeen main spices found in the Indian spice cabinet and their merits:

1. **Turmeric** (*haldi*): It is rich in antioxidants and can help fight cancer due to the main component—*curcumin*. This spice helps minimize liver disease, arthritis, and joint inflammation. It is an antiseptic and antibacterial—disinfects cuts/wounds and treats skin infections. It reduces cholesterol and aids in fat metabolism, resulting in weight reduction. Turmeric prevents the growth of new blood vessels in tumors and reduces the risk of childhood leukemia. *Note: Turmeric should not be used by those who are suffering from gallstones or bile obstruction, without first consulting a doctor or an Ayurvedacharya. Also, while using this spice, please be careful, since it can leave stains (e.g., on kitchen counters).*

2. **Black pepper** (*kali mirch*): It improves the digestion of food upon reaching the stomach, facilitates the stimulation of hydrochloric acid in the stomach, which helps reduce intestinal gas, and prevents bacterial growth in the intestine. The spice is also known to increase appetite and would be helpful to those suffering from anorexia. The antibacterial properties are evident when used over a cut to stop the bleeding. It acts as a diuretic and encourages our body to sweat and remove toxins. The outer shell of the whole peppercorn breaks down fat cells and can help reduce weight. It relieves joint pain, can prevent earaches, treats toothaches, and breaks up cold congestion. Black

pepper is a source of manganese, potassium, iron, vitamins C and K, and dietary fiber. *Note: Black pepper should not be consumed by those suffering with ulcers or those who have undergone abdominal surgery, without first consulting a doctor or Ayurvedacharya.*

3. **Asafoetida** (*hing*): It assists in the treatment of respiratory issues such as asthma, bronchitis, and whooping cough. If mixed in water, it can be consumed for relieving headaches and migraines. In addition, this spice assists in dealing with depression and mood swings. Asafoetida is a carminative that aids in proper digestion. It provides great protection against bad cholesterol and triglycerides. It is good for treating impotence in men and painful or excessive menstruation in women. The sedative properties help lower blood pressure.

4. **Red chili** (*lal mirchi*): **powder** This contains capsaicin which is effective not only in the treatment of stomach ulcers, but also boosts metabolism and immunity in the body. It helps to remove congestion from the nose and lungs. Red Chili powder is good for the treatment of sensory nerve fiber issues.

5. **Cumin** (*jeera*): Improves appetite and can be used for many digestive disorders, such as indigestion, flatulence, and diarrhea. It increases metabolism, speeds up the liver detoxification process, and balances the Tridoshas in the body, resulting in improved health. It is effective in reducing nausea associated with pregnancy. It is an antiseptic that can relieve the symptoms of sore throat and colds, and consuming roasted cumin will remove bad breath. Cumin seeds contain a good amount of iron, which is beneficial for anemia and for stimulating the menstrual cycle.

6. **Coriander** (*dhania*): Coriander improves appetite, is good for digestion, lowers blood sugar, and regulates insulin levels. Dry coriander helps cure diarrhea. This spice acts as a natural diuretic and helps the body discharge water/urine. It helps in curing fever, inflammation, certain allergies, and calms tired eyes. It is effective in restoring Pitta balance due to its cooling effects and is used to cure sunstroke in the summer months. The antiseptic, antifungal, and disinfectant properties contained in coriander are used in the treatment of dry skin, eczema, other skin disorders, and small pox.

7. **Clove** (*launga*): Cloves are a natural anesthetic that can be used for toothaches and to fight arthritis pain. Clove oil helps with blood circulation and stimulates the skin upon application, making it beneficial for acne. It reduces flatulence and nausea, promotes digestion, boosts memory, and is beneficial for the heart, liver, and stomach.
8. **Saffron** (*kesar*): This spice has an aromatic smell that enhances the taste of food and is used quite commonly in Indian desserts. It improves appetite and digestion. Saffron is used in the treatment of kidney/bladder/liver disorders, improves memory, enhances vision, and lightens the skin tone. Saffron tea can be used to treat depression.
9. **Cinnamon** (*dalchini*): It improves memory, appetite, and digestion. Cinnamon is known to treat diabetes – it can lower LDL cholesterol and blood sugar levels. This spice provides significant relief for arthritis pain in the joints, and aids with migraines. It reduces headaches pain, mental stress, and body temperature during a fever.
10. **Cardamom** (*elaichi*): Cardamom helps with bad breath, nausea, stomach acidity, flatulence, and the inherent detoxifying properties aid in cleansing the body. It increases appetite, improves overall digestion, and balances the Tridoshas. Cardamom is a well-known aphrodisiac.
11. **Fenugreek** (*methi*): Fenugreek restores healthy cholesterol levels and reduces blood sugar levels in diabetics. It has a soothing effect on the digestive organs and reduces gastric inflammation, reflux, and heartburn. It helps in treating constipation and suppresses the appetite. Fenugreek relieves skin inflammation—boils, burns, and eczema. It aids in reducing fever and flu symptoms (sore throat and cough), eases anxiety, insomnia, and menopause.
12. **Ginger** (*adrak*): Fresh ginger is effective in the treatment of morning motion sickness, migraines, heartburn, cold, flu, and asthma. It is a carminative that promotes the elimination of intestinal gas. Regular intake of ginger will reduce the pain of rheumatoid arthritis. It is an antiseptic and antifungal, promotes sweating, and increases blood flow.

7. **Garlic** (*lasoon*): Regular intake can lower blood pressure, control blood sugar, and boost immunity. It detoxifies and cleanses the body. Garlic is good for coughs, throat infections and reduces the severity of upper-respiratory-tract infections. It is a natural antioxidant that protects against bacterial and viral infections. This will help to thin the blood which aids in the prevention of heart disease.
8. **Curry leaf:** Curry leaves have antioxidant, anti-inflammatory properties that can help restore the skin when applied on cuts, bruises, burns, and insect bites. This spice helps with stress and diarrhea. The application of a mixture of hair oil and curry leaf on the scalp is beneficial in strengthening hair roots.
9. **Bay leaf** (*tejpatta*): It contains copper, potassium, vitamin C, calcium, magnesium, and iron. Bay leaf is used in the treatment of diabetes, colic pain, abdominal pain, bacterial and fungal infections, colds, migraines, high blood pressure, and respiratory and urinary tract infections.
10. **Mustard seed** (*rai*): It contains *selenium*, which can reduce the severity of asthma, rheumatoid arthritis, the frequency of migraines, and the effect of cancer. Mustard seeds are a good source of zinc, omega-3s, iron, calcium, manganese, and dietary fiber. It improves digestion and increases metabolism.
11. **Nutmeg** (*jaiphal*): Nutmeg is an anti-inflammatory, which can provide relief from joint pain. Powdered nutmeg in water will provide relief from menstrual cramps. It offers relief from diarrhea, constipation, flatulence, and bloating. The antibacterial properties help fight bad breath and can be used to treat gum disease or toothaches. It is used to remove toxins, dissolve kidney stones, and detox the liver and kidneys. This flavorful spice not only boosts appetite but also induces sleep.

Chapter 11
Food Charts and Quantification

Ayurveda advises that you must eat the quantity of food that is right for your stomach size and be satisfied, without overeating. The stomach should be filled in accordance with this formula – one-third with solid food, one-third with liquid, and keep one-third empty. Water can be consumed during the meal; drinking warm or room temperature water prior to each meal is suggested.

The ancient science of Ayurveda followed a measurement method using the palm of the hand. Ayurveda states that the adequate meal size per person (*serving size 1*) should be that of an *Anjali*, or *the quantity that fits the two cupped palms held close together*. The liquid was measured by holding the liquid in the palm of the hand. The measurements for the raw ingredients / food items below have been arrived at by using a measurement method to quantify the amount held in one closed fist (of a medium-structured adult).

Name of Food	Measurement
Root Vegetables:	
Beetroot	¾ cup
Carrot	¾ cup
Horseradish	¾ cup
Jicama	½ cup
Onions	¾ cup
Parsnip	½ cup
Potato	½ cup
Radish	¾ cup
Ratalu	½ cup
Sweet potato	½ cup
Turnip	½ cup
Yam	½ cup
Yucca	½ cup

Stem Vegetables:

Asparagus	10–12 (1" pieces)
Celery	12–15 (1" pieces)
Leek	14–16 (1" pieces)
Pearl onions	10–12 (1" pieces)
Rhubarb	8–10 (1" pieces)
Scallion	14–16 (1" pieces)

Leafy Vegetables:

Alfalfa sprouts	1 cup
Amaranth leaves	1 cup
Arugula	1 cup
Basil	1 cup
Broccoli rabe	1 cup
Bok choy	1 cup
Collard greens	1 cup
Dandelion greens	1 cup
Fenugreek leaves	1 cup
Grape leaves	1 cup
Kale	1 cup
Lettuce	1 cup
Mustard greens	1 cup
Napa cabbage	1 cup
Spinach	1 cup
Swiss chard	1 cup
Watercress	1 cup

Flower Vegetables:

Artichokes	8–10 pieces
Broccoli	10–14 (1" pieces)
Brussel sprouts	8–9 pieces
Cabbage	1 cup (shredded/thin slivers)
Cauliflower	10–14 (1" pieces)

Fruit Vegetables:

Avocado	1 cup
Bell pepper	1 cup
Bitter gourd	1 cup
Bottle gourd	1 cup
Cucumber	1 cup
Eggplant	1 cup
Snake gourd / parval	1 cup
Pumpkin	¾ cup
Olives	¾ cup
Squash	¾ cup
Sun-dried tomato	¾ cup
Sweet corn	1 cup
Tomato	1 cup
Apple gourd / tinda	1 cup
Zucchini	1 cup

Podded Vegetables:

Cluster beans	½ cup
Drumstick	6–8 (1" pieces)
Green beans	8–10 (1" pieces)
Okra	20–25 (1" pieces)
Peas	⅓ cup
Pigeon peas	½ cup
Runner beans	10–12 (1" pieces)
Snow peas	⅓ cup

Nuts (if eaten alone):

Almonds (with skin)	12–14 pieces
Almonds (soaked, peeled)	13–15 pieces
Brazil nuts	5–6 pieces
Cashews	6–8 pieces
Chestnuts	8–10 pieces
Coconut	5–6 (1" pieces)
Hazelnuts	8–10 pieces
Macadamia nuts	8–10 pieces
Peanuts	10–12 pieces
Pecans (no shell)	8–10 pieces
Pistachios (no shell)	10 pieces
Pine nuts	⅛ cup
Walnuts	8–10 pieces

Seeds (if eaten alone):

Chia seeds	¼ cup
Hemp seeds	⅓ cup
Flaxseed	¼ cup
Pumpkin seeds	⅛ cup
Safflower seeds	⅛ cup
Sesame seeds	¼ cup
Sunflower seeds	⅛ cup

Grains:

Amaranth	¼ cup
Bajra	¼ cup
Barley	¼ cup
Brown rice	¼ cup
Bulghur	¼ cup
Buckwheat	¼ cup
Corn	⅛ cup
Cream of wheat	¼ cup
Farro	¼ cup

Food Charts and Quantification

Jowar	¼ cup
Kamut	¼ cup
Millet	¼ cup
Oats/oatmeal	¼ cup
Quinoa	¼ cup
Basmati rice	¼ cup
Rye	¼ cup
Rolled oats	¼ cup
Sago/tapioca	⅛ cup
Spelt	⅛ cup
Teff	¼ cup
Wheat bran	¼ cup
Whole wheat flour	⅓ cup

Dairy:

Almond milk	¼ cup with oatmeal / 8 ounces if it is consumed alone
Buffalo's milk	¼ cup with oatmeal / 8 ounces if it is consumed alone
Butter	¼ teaspoon
Buttermilk	8 ounces
Cheese	1 tablespoon
Cottage cheese	4–6 ounces
Cow's milk	¼ cup with oatmeal / 8 ounces if it is consumed alone
Egg whites	3 (plain—with no additions)
Eggs with yolk	1
Frozen yogurt	4–6 ounces
Ghee	½ teaspoon
Goat's milk	¼ cup with oatmeal / 8 ounces if it is consumed alone
Greek yogurt	4-6 ounces
Ice cream	4 ounces
Low-fat milk	½ cup with oatmeal / 8 ounces if it is consumed alone

Rice milk	½ cup with oatmeal / 8 ounces if it is consumed alone
Skim milk	½ cup with oatmeal / 8 ounces if it is consumed alone
Soy yogurt	4–6 ounces
Sour cream	1 tablespoon
Tofu	½ cup
Whipped cream	1 tablespoon
Whole milk	¼ cup with oatmeal / 8 ounces if it is consumed alone
Yogurt (homemade)	4–6 ounces

Sweeteners:

Barley malt syrup	¼ teaspoon
Brown sugar	¼ teaspoon
Date sugar	¼ teaspoon
Honey	¼ teaspoon
Jaggery	¼ teaspoon
Maple syrup	¼ teaspoon
Misri (crystallized sugar)	¼ teaspoon
Sugar	¼ teaspoon

Beans and Legumes:

Adzuki beans	¼ cup
Black beans	¼ cup
Black-eyed peas	¼ cup
Black lentils	¼ cup
Cannellini beans	¼ cup
Chickpeas	¼ cup
Fava beans	¼ cup
Kidney beans	¼ cup
Lentils	¼ cup
Lima beans	¼ cup
Mung beans	¼ cup

Navy beans	¼ cup
Pink beans	¼ cup
Pinto beans	¼ cup
Red gram	¼ cup
Soy beans	¼ cup
Urad dal	¼ cup
Yellow lentils	¼ cup

Nonvegetarian:

Beef	¼ cup
Chicken	⅓ cup (3 ounces, depending on thickness, or half a breast)
Duck	⅓ cup (3 ounces, depending on thickness, of half a breast)
Fish	½ cup (4 ounces of 1" thickness)
Shrimp/tuna	⅓ cup
Lamb	⅓ cup
Pork	¼ cup
Turkey	⅓ cup (thin slices)

Oils:

Almond oil	¼ tablespoon
Corn oil	¼ tablespoon
Coconut oil	⅛ tablespoon
Ghee	⅛ tablespoon
Mustard oil	⅛ tablespoon
Olive oil	¼ tablespoon
Peanut oil	¼ tablespoon
Safflower oil	¼ tablespoon
Sesame oil	¼ tablespoon
Sunflower oil	¼ tablespoon
Vegetable oil	¼ tablespoon

Spices:

Ajwain / carom seed	⅛ teaspoon
Asafoetida	⅛ teaspoon
Basil	1–2 leaves
Bay leaves	1 medium leaf
Black pepper	¼ teaspoon
Black salt	⅛ teaspoon
Cardamom	¼ teaspoon
Cinnamon	⅛ teaspoon
Cloves	1–2 pieces
Coriander powder	¼ teaspoon
Cumin	¼ teaspoon
Curry leaves	1–2 leaves
Dill	⅛ teaspoon
Fennel	⅛ teaspoon
Fenugreek	2–4 leaves
Garlic	½ pod
Ginger (fresh)	¼" piece
Ginger powder (dry)	⅛ teaspoon
Green chilies	1 piece
Kokum	1 piece
Lemon juice	¼ teaspoon
Mint	⅛ teaspoon
Mustard seeds	⅛ teaspoon
Nutmeg	⅛ teaspoon
Red chili powder	¼ teaspoon
Rock salt	⅛ teaspoon
Rosemary	⅛ teaspoon
Saffron	⅛ teaspoon
Sea salt	⅛ teaspoon
Tamarind	¼ teaspoon
Thyme	⅛ teaspoon
Turmeric powder	¼ teaspoon

Chapter 12
Daily Intake Chart by Constitution

(Note: The calorie chart below is for those who would like to know the amount of calories that can be consumed on a daily basis as per their specific constitution. However, Ayurveda does not follow the calorie charts in determining the size of the meals. The focus is placed on the quality of the food and the quality of Agni, which aids in the digestive process.)

Please be advised that the calorie ranges below have been established with guidance from a fitness trainer and an Ayurvedacharya.

Meals	Vata		Pitta		Kapha	
Activity Level	Low	High	Low	High	Low	High
Total Calorie Range	*1,800 calories*	*2,000 calories*	*1,600 calories*	*1,800 calories*	*1,300 calories*	*1,600 calories*
Breakfast	500 calories	500 calories	300 calories	400 calories	300 calories	400 calories
Snack	200 calories	200 calories	200 calories	200 calories	150 calories	150 calories
Lunch	500 calories	600 calories	500 calories	500 calories	400 calories	500 calories
Snack	200 calories	200 calories	200 calories	200 calories	150 calories	250 calories
Dinner	400 calories	500 calories	400 calories	500 calories	300 calories	300 calories

Chapter 13
Recipes

Broccoli with Butter
Good for doshas: Vata and Kapha
Serving size: 1

Ingredients:
10–15 broccoli florets
1 cup of water
¼ tablespoon unsalted butter
Salt to taste
Black pepper to taste

Method:
1. Cut or separate the broccoli florets into 1" wide pieces. Put the broccoli in a pot with 1 cup of water and bring to a boil. Cover and cook over medium heat for 5 minutes or until tender. Drain the extra water.
2. Add the butter, salt, and black pepper to taste. Mix thoroughly and serve.

Saffron Basmati Rice
Good for doshas: all doshas
Serving size: 1

Ingredients:
¼ cup brown basmati rice
¾ cup boiling water
A pinch of salt
2 strands of saffron
⅛ tablespoon ghee

Method:
1. In a pot, add the rice, water, salt, and saffron.
2. Cover and simmer over a low heat for 40 minutes. Remove from the heat, mix in the ghee, and serve hot.

Chicken Curry

Good for doshas: all doshas
Serving size: 1

Ingredients:
¾ tablespoon coconut oil
¼ teaspoon cumin seeds
½ cinnamon stick
1 cardamom
1 clove
¼ teaspoon fresh ginger, chopped finely
1 small green chili, chopped finely
⅛ teaspoon garlic, chopped finely
½ onion, chopped finely
¼ teaspoon turmeric powder
½ tablespoon dhania-jeera powder
½ tablespoon fresh tomato paste
Salt to taste
½ cup hot water
½–1 skinless chicken breast, cut into small pieces
¼ tomato, chopped finely
¼ tablespoon fresh cream (preferable to avoid)
¾ tablespoon cilantro, chopped finely for the garnish

Method:
1. In a large pot on a medium flame, add ¼ tablespoon oil, cumin seeds, cinnamon, cardamom, clove, ginger, green chilies, garlic, onions and sauté until the onions become translucent.
2. Add the turmeric dhania-jeera powder and sauté gently for 5 minutes.
3. Put in the tomato paste, salt, and hot water. Bring to a boil. Simmer for 20 minutes.
4. In a separate pan, add ½ tablespoon oil, add the chicken pieces, and stir-fry until they turn white.
5. Add the cooked chicken and tomatoes to the gravy and simmer until the meat becomes succulent. Add the cream.
6. Garnish with chopped cilantro and serve hot.

Moong and Spinach Dal

Good for doshas: all doshas
Serving size: 1

Ingredients:
½ cup whole moong
1 cup of water
½ cup chopped spinach
½ teaspoon cumin seeds
¼ teaspoon mustard seeds
½ tablespoon dried coconut
1 tablespoon urad dal
¼ teaspoon turmeric powder
¼ teaspoon black pepper
Salt to taste

Method:
1. Wash and soak the whole moong for 2 hours. Drain and put in a deep pot of boiling water (1 cup). Cook for 15–20 minutes. Add in the chopped spinach and cook for 5–8 minutes.
2. In a separate pan, dry-roast the cumin seeds, mustard seeds, coconut, urad dal, turmeric powder, black pepper, and salt. Add to the moong dal and spinach mixture. Cook for 30 minutes until soft.
3. Add water if you want to make it like a soup, or serve it thick and hot.

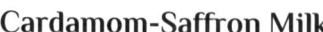

Cardamom-Saffron Milk

Good for doshas: Vata
Serving size: 1

Ingredients:
1 cup skim milk
¼ teaspoon cardamom powder
4 strands of saffron
¼ teaspoon honey

Method:
1. In a pot, boil the milk. Add the cardamom powder and saffron strands.
2. Pour in a cup and add the honey. Drink hot.

Banana and Fenugreek Leaves

Good for doshas: Vata and Pitta
Serving size: 1

Ingredients:
¼ cup banana
1 cup fenugreek leaves
⅛ tablespoon ghee
¼ teaspoon mustard seeds
¼ teaspoon asafoetida
¼ teaspoon chopped green chilies
¼ teaspoon chopped ginger
⅛ teaspoon turmeric powder
⅛ teaspoon garam masala powder
2 tablespoons lemon juice
¾ tablespoon cilantro, chopped finely for the garnish
Salt to taste

Method:
1. Peel and chop the bananas into small pieces.
2. Chop the fenugreek leaves.
3. In a saucepan, add the ghee and mustard seeds. When they pop, add the asafoetida and fenugreek leaves.
4. Add salt and cook until the leaves soften.
5. Add the green chilies, ginger, turmeric powder, garam masala powder, banana pieces and stir well.
6. Sprinkle in the lemon juice, mix, garnish with chopped cilantro, and serve hot.

Dry Fruit Smoothie

Good for doshas: all doshas
Serving size: 1

Ingredients:
5–8 raisins
1 tablespoon dates, chopped finely
4–5 prunes, chopped
½ cup water
½ cup almond milk

Method:
1. Put all the ingredients in a blender and blend for a few minutes until semismooth. Serve.

Brown Rice Khicchadi

Good for doshas: all doshas
Serving size: 1

Ingredients:
¼ cup whole moong dal
¼ cup brown basmati rice
⅛ tablespoon ghee
¼ teaspoon black peppercorns
¼ teaspoon cumin seeds
1 cup boiling water
A pinch of salt
A pinch of turmeric powder

Method:
1. Soak the moong dal in 1 cup of water at room temperature for 2 hours and drain. Wash the rice and dal until the water becomes clear.
2. In a large, deep pot, heat the ghee and sauté the peppercorns and cumin seeds.
3. Add the rice and dal. Sauté over low heat for 3 minutes.
4. Add the boiling water, salt, and turmeric powder.
5. Cover and simmer over a low heat for 1 hour, stirring to prevent it from burning. Serve warm.

Quinoa with Carrots

Good for doshas: all doshas
Serving size: 1

Ingredients:
½ cup quinoa
¾ cup water
¼ cup carrots, chopped finely
A pinch of salt

Method:
1. Wash the quinoa. In a pot, add the water and carrots. Bring to a boil.
2. Add the quinoa and salt. Cover and simmer over a low heat for 15–20 minutes. Serve hot.

Leek-Flavored Quinoa

Good for doshas: all doshas
Serving size: 1

Ingredients:
1 leek
⅛ tablespoon ghee
¼ teaspoon cumin seeds
¼ cup prerinsed quinoa
¾ cup water

Method:
1. Cut the leek into small pieces.
2. In a pan, heat the ghee, add the cumin seeds. When lightly brown, add the leek and sauté.
3. Put in the prerinsed quinoa, add the water, and bring to a simmer.
4. Reduce the gas heat to low and cook for 35 minutes.
5. Remove from heat and let it sit for 5 minutes.
6. Fluff and serve.

Whole Moong Dal

Good for doshas: Vata and Kapha
Serving size: 1

Ingredients:
½ cup whole moong dal
1 cup water
¼ teaspoon coriander powder
⅛ teaspoon turmeric powder
⅛ tablespoon ghee
¼ teaspoon cumin seeds
¼ teaspoon grated fresh ginger
¼ green chili, chopped finely
¼ teaspoon lemon juice
¾ tablespoon cilantro, chopped finely for the garnish
A pinch of salt
A pinch of asafoetida

Method:
1. Soak the whole moong dal in water overnight. Drain.
2. Boil 1 cup of water, add the moong dal, salt, asafoetida, coriander powder, and turmeric powder. Simmer over a medium heat for 45 minutes.
3. In a separate pan, add the ghee, cumin seeds, ginger, and green chili. Sauté for a couple of minutes.
4. Add the spice mixture to the dal, cover, and simmer over a low heat for another 20 minutes. Add the lemon juice, garnish with chopped cilantro, and serve hot.

Mint Lassi (Buttermilk)

Good for doshas: Vata and Pitta
Serving size: 1

Ingredients:
¼ teaspoon ground cumin seeds
4 ounces plain yogurt
¼ teaspoon chopped, fresh mint leaves
1 cup water
Salt to taste
Black pepper to taste
A couple of cilantro leaves for garnish

Method:
1. In a flat pan, dry-roast the ground cumin seeds and black pepper while stirring constantly, until the aroma is released.
2. Combine the cumin seeds, yogurt, mint leaves, water, salt, and pepper in a blender.
3. Garnish with cilantro leaves.
4. Serve cold.

Carrot and Broccoli Soup

Good for doshas: Kapha
Serving size: 1

Ingredients:
2 cups water
½ cup sliced carrots
1 cup broccoli florets
¼ cup sliced onions
¼ teaspoon of fresh, chopped ginger
½ teaspoon coriander powder
¼ teaspoon turmeric powder
Salt to taste

Method:
1. In a deep pot, boil the water. Add the carrots, broccoli, onions, ginger, salt, coriander powder, and turmeric powder.
2. Boil on a low heat for about 30 minutes. Serve hot.

Garlic-Flavored Potatoes

Good for doshas: Pitta
Serving size: 1

Ingredients:
¾ cup Yukon potatoes
1½ cups water
¼ teaspoon fresh garlic, chopped finely
¼ tablespoon unsalted butter
1 tablespoon milk
Salt to taste
Black pepper to taste

Method:
1. Put the potatoes in a pot, then cover with water. Bring to a boil, reduce the heat, and boil for 5–10 minutes until tender.
2. Strain the water, mash, add butter and garlic. Mix thoroughly. Add the milk and mix again.
3. Add the salt and black pepper to taste, mix, and serve.

Kale Chips

Good for doshas: Pitta and Kapha
Serving size: 1

Ingredients:
1 bunch of fresh kale
¼ tablespoon olive oil
Salt to taste
Black pepper / red chili powder to taste

Method:
1. Wash the kale and separate the leaves.
2. Preheat the oven to 350 degrees Fahrenheit and arrange the leaves in a baking tray.
3. Sprinkle the olive oil on the kale leaves.
4. Bake for 5–10 minutes until crisp (the leaves should not become brown).
5. Remove the tray and cool.
6. Sprinkle with salt and black pepper or red chili powder as per your taste.

Recipes

Gram Flour Pancake

Good for doshas: all doshas
Serving size: 1

Ingredients:
½ cup gram flour (besan)
¼ bunch fresh spinach, washed and chopped finely
¼ onion, chopped finely
¼ teaspoon fresh ginger, minced
¼ teaspoon red chili powder
¼ tablespoon cilantro, chopped finely
¼ teaspoon turmeric powder
¼ cup water
½ tablespoon olive oil
1 teaspoon flax seeds
Salt to taste

Method:
1. In a bowl, mix the gram flour, flax seeds, spinach, onion, ginger, salt, red chili powder, cilantro, and turmeric powder. Add water and make a medium-thick batter.
2. Heat a flat skillet on a low flame; when the skillet is warm, add olive oil, a dollop of the gram flour batter, and spread quickly to form a pancake.
3. Flip the pancake on the other side and cook until golden brown. Serve hot.

Couscous and Carrots

Good for doshas: Vata and Pitta
Serving size: 1

Ingredients:
¾ cup water
¼ cup couscous
⅛ cup finely chopped carrots
1 tablespoon chopped cilantro

Method:
1. Bring water to boil in a pot; add the couscous and carrots.
2. Cover and simmer on low heat for 5–10 minutes.
3. Garnish with chopped cilantro and serve.

Roasted Butternut Squash Soup

Good for doshas: all doshas
Serving size: 1

Ingredients:
½ cup butternut squash
¼ apple
¼ cup onion
1 cup vegetable broth
Salt to taste
Black pepper to taste
Green chili-ginger paste to taste
¼ teaspoon nutmeg powder
2–3 fresh mint leaves

Method:
1. Cut the butternut squash, apple, and onion into 1" pieces.
2. Put the vegetable broth, onion, apple, and butternut squash pieces in a pot, cover, and bring to a boil.
3. Reduce to low-medium heat, uncover, and let the mixture simmer for 10 minutes.
4. Puree the soup. Add the salt, black pepper, green chili-ginger paste, and nutmeg powder.
5. Garnish with the mint leaves. Serve hot or cold.

Note: Green chili-ginger paste can be made by grinding about 4 green chilies (remove the stems) and a 1" piece of fresh ginger in an electric grinder.

Adzuki Beans

Good for doshas: Pitta and Kapha
Serving size: 1

Ingredients:
¼ cup adzuki beans
1½ cups water
A pinch of salt
⅛ tablespoon ghee
⅛ teaspoon black mustard seeds
¼ cup shallots, chopped in thin slivers
¼ teaspoon turmeric powder
¼ teaspoon lemon juice
¾ tablespoon cilantro, chopped finely

Method:
1. Soak the adzuki beans overnight. Drain and rinse.
2. In a large, deep pot, bring the adzuki beans to a boil in 1½ cups of water.
3. Cover and simmer over medium heat for 1 hour.
4. In a separate pan, add the ghee, mustard seeds, and when they pop, add the shallots. Sauté the shallots for a few minutes, then add the turmeric powder and salt.
5. Add the beans, cover, and simmer over a low heat for 30–35 minutes. Remove from heat, add the lemon juice, garnish with chopped cilantro, and serve warm.

Chicken Salad

Good for doshas: all doshas
Serving size: 1

Ingredients:
½ medium tomato, chopped finely
½ onion, chopped finely
1 green chili, chopped finely
¼ teaspoon fresh ginger, chopped finely
¼ cucumber, chopped finely
¼ teaspoon curry powder
¼ tablespoon olive oil
½ tablespoon lemon juice
⅓–¼ cup chicken, cooked and shredded
¾ cup romaine lettuce, chopped in thin slivers
Salt to taste
¾ tablespoon cilantro, chopped finely for the garnish
½ tablespoon almonds, sliced finely and roasted, for the garnish

Method:
1. In a large mixing bowl, add the tomatoes, onions, green chili, ginger, and cucumber. To this mixture, add in salt, curry powder, olive oil, and lemon juice. Mix well.
2. Add in the chicken pieces to the salad mixture.
3. In a serving dish, make a bed of lettuce. Put the chicken salad mixture on the lettuce.
4. Garnish with cilantro and roasted almonds and serve.

Cooked Beets

Good for doshas: Vata and Kapha
Serving size: 1

Ingredients:
⅛ tablespoon ghee
1 dry red chili
1 bay leaf
⅛ teaspoon mustard seeds
¼ teaspoon cumin seeds
¾ cup chopped red beetroots (steamed)
½ green chili, chopped finely
¼ teaspoon chopped, fresh ginger
¼ teaspoon chopped, fresh cilantro/coriander
¼ teaspoon fresh lemon juice
Salt to taste
Pomegranate seeds for the garnish

Method:
1. In a saucepan, heat the ghee. Add the dry red chili, bay leaf, and mustard seeds.
2. When the mustard seeds start to pop, add the cumin seeds. When they are light brown, add the beets, salt, green chilies, and ginger. Cook until the beetroot pieces are soft.
3. Remove from heat and mix with the cilantro and lemon juice.
4. Garnish with pomegranate seeds and serve.

Cooked Radish

Good for doshas: Kapha
Serving size: 1

Ingredients:
⅛ tablespoon ghee
1 dry red chili
1 bay leaf
⅛ teaspoon mustard seeds
¼ teaspoon cumin seeds
¾ cup chopped radish
½ green chili, chopped finely
¼ teaspoon fresh lemon juice
¼ teaspoon chopped, fresh ginger
Salt to taste
¼ teaspoon chopped, fresh cilantro/coriander, for the garnish

Method:
1. In a saucepan, heat the ghee. Add the dry red chili, bay leaf, and mustard seeds.
2. When the mustard seeds start to pop, add the cumin seeds. When they are light brown, add the radish, salt, green chili, and ginger, cover, and cook until the radish pieces are soft.
3. Remove from heat, mix in the cilantro/coriander and lemon juice. Serve.

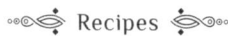 Recipes

Steamed Cauliflower, Carrots, and Broccoli

Good for doshas: Pitta and Kapha
Serving size: 1

Ingredients:
1 cup broccoli florets
½ cup chopped carrot (1" pieces)
8–10 florets of cauliflower
Salt to taste

Method:
1. Place all three vegetables in a steamer and cook or steam for 10 minutes. Sprinkle a pinch of salt on the steamed vegetables and serve hot.

Cumin Quinoa

Good for doshas: all doshas
Serving size: 1

Ingredients:
½ cup quinoa
¾ cup water
¼ tablespoon cumin seeds
A pinch of turmeric powder
A pinch of salt

Method:
1. Wash the quinoa. In a pot, add the water and salt and bring to a boil.
2. In a separate pan, dry-roast the cumin seeds and turmeric powder. Add to the water.
3. Add the quinoa, cover, and simmer over a low heat for another 5 minutes. Serve hot.

Bajra Rotla (Millet Bread)

Good for doshas: Kapha
Serving size: 1

Ingredients:
¼ cup millet flour
⅛ tablespoon ghee
¼ cup warm water
Salt to taste

Method:
1. Mix the flour and salt together in a bowl.
2. Rub ghee into the flour and mix.
3. Add warm water to form the dough.
4. Take some dough in your hand and form a small ball.
5. With wet palms, flatten the ball into a 6" even round.
6. Heat a *tava* / flat pan on medium heat and put the round *rotla* on it.
7. Turn each side and cook until small brown spots appear.
8. Serve hot with spicy vegetables.

Corn Khicchadi

Good for doshas: Kapha
Serving size: 1

Ingredients:
2 fresh whole corn cobs
¼ tablespoon olive oil
¼ teaspoon mustard seeds
¼ teaspoon cumin seeds
¼ teaspoon chopped green chilies
¼ teaspoon chopped fresh ginger
⅛ teaspoon turmeric powder
¼ cup water
½ teaspoon lemon juice
¼ tablespoon chopped cilantro/coriander leaves, for the garnish
Salt to taste

Method:
1. Peel and grate the corn in a bowl.
2. In a saucepan, put in the oil, mustard seeds, cumin seeds, green chilies, ginger, and turmeric powder.
3. When the mustard seeds pop, add the corn and cook for 10 minutes.
4. Add the water and salt. Cover and cook until the corn is tender.
5. Add lemon juice and mix.
6. Garnish with cilantro/coriander and serve hot.

Adai (Moong Dal Pancake)

Good for doshas: all doshas
Serving size: 1

Ingredients:

¼ cup whole moong dal
½ cup water
1 dry curry leaf
⅛ cup brown basmati or millet
¼ teaspoon fresh ginger, chopped finely
¼ teaspoon green chili, chopped finely
½ tablespoon cilantro, chopped finely
A pinch of salt
⅛ tablespoon ghee
¼ tablespoon olive oil

Method:

1. Soak the moong dal and rice separately in about 2"–3" of water overnight.
2. Rinse and drain the moong dal, put it in a food processor, and grind it with the curry leaf to a rough, coarse-textured paste. Set aside.
3. Rinse and drain the rice, put it in a food processor, and grind it to a rough, coarse-textured paste.
4. Combine the two mixtures; add in the ginger, green chili, cilantro, salt, and ghee.
5. Add a few tablespoons of water to form a thick batter.
6. Heat a pancake griddle and coat with a thin film of olive oil.
7. Spread the batter to form a pancake about ¼" thick and as large as the size of the pancake griddle pan.
8. Cook for 3–4 minutes on each side over medium heat. Serve hot with a spiced yogurt or chutney.

Dessert Options

Chocolate and Nut Cups
Good for doshas: Vata and Kapha
Serving size: 1

Ingredients:
2 ounces melted bittersweet chocolate
1 tablespoon pistachio pieces
1 tablespoon walnut pieces
¼ tablespoon pumpkin seeds
½ tablespoon dried cherries
½ tablespoon golden raisins
2 fresh mint leaves, finely chopped

Method:
1. Pour the melted chocolate into 4 paper/foil cups (1.5" × 1" deep), filling them with ¼ inch of chocolate in each.
2. On top of the soft chocolate, arrange the pistachios, walnuts, pumpkin seeds, cherries, raisins, and mint leaves and press lightly to embed into the chocolate.
3. Refrigerate for 1 hour until they harden.
4. Remove the cups from the papers/foils and arrange on a plate. Serve and enjoy.

Pear Crumble

Good for doshas: all doshas
Serving size: 1

Ingredients:
1½ pears
¼ teaspoon honey
½ tablespoon oats

Method:
1. Chop the pears into long pieces.
2. Preheat the oven to 300 degrees Fahrenheit.
3. Put the pear in an oven-safe pan and add honey.
4. Sprinkle the oats on top and cook for 5–10 minutes.
5. Remove and serve warm.

Suji (Semolina) Halwa

Good for doshas: Vata and Pitta
Serving size: 1

Ingredients:
⅛ tablespoon ghee
¼ cup suji (semolina)
1 cup water
1 tablespoon milk
1 teaspoon brown sugar
6 raisins
¼ teaspoon cardamom powder

Method:
1. In a saucepan, heat the ghee, add the semolina, and roast until it turns light brown in color.
2. Remove from the pan and put aside.
3. Combine 1 cup water, milk, brown sugar, raisins, and cardamom powder.
4. Mix and bring to a boil.
5. Add the roasted semolina; mix until the liquid dries and the mixture becomes thick.
6. Serve hot.

Amaranth-Jaggery Sweet

Good for doshas: all doshas
Serving size: 1

Ingredients:
¼ cup amaranth flour
1 tablespoon ghee
1 tablespoon milk
⅛ cup jaggery slivers (thin strips)
¼ teaspoon cardamom powder

Method:
1. In a saucepan, stir the amaranth flour with ghee until slightly light brown.
2. Add the milk and cook for another five minutes.
3. Remove from heat. While the mixture is hot, add the jaggery slivers and mix well.
4. Pour onto a metal plate (preferably steel) and allow it to set.
5. Sprinkle the cardamom powder, cut into pieces, and store in an airtight container. Enjoy!

Chocolate-Covered Raisins

Good for doshas: Kapha
Serving size: 1

Ingredients:
⅛ slab of organic dark chocolate (4-ounce bar, 70% cocoa content or above)
A pinch of red chili powder
10 raisins

Method:
1. Melt the dark chocolate in a pot in hot water on the stove. Add the red chili powder and stir.
2. Put in the raisins in the chocolate syrup to cover completely.
3. Remove and spread out on a baking tray. Chill for about 45 minutes and serve.

Almond-Date Cake

Good for doshas: all doshas
Serving size: 1

Ingredients:
5–6 pieces of blanched almonds
5 pitted dates
¼ teaspoon almond extract
¼ cup almond milk
¾ cup barley flour
¼ cup water
A pinch of salt
A pinch of baking soda

Method:
1. Preheat oven to 350 degrees Fahrenheit.
2. Using a food processor, puree the almonds, dates, almond extract, and almond milk into a cream-like consistency.
3. In a bowl, combine the barley flour, salt, baking soda, and pureed mixture.
4. Add water and knead into a batter.
5. Pour the batter into a greased baking dish and bake for 30 minutes. Serve.

Peanut Brittle or Chikki

Good for doshas: Vata
Serving size: 1 plate of chikki (can be cut into 1" × 1" squares/pieces)

Ingredients:
½ pound peanuts
1 tablespoon sesame seeds
½ cup water
1 pound jaggery or gur
½ teaspoon cardamom powder
1 tablespoon ghee

Method:
1. Dry-roast the peanuts and put aside to cool. Then crush in a food processor or blender for a couple of minutes, to form a coarse powder with small pieces. Dry-roast the sesame seeds separately and set them aside too.
2. In a pan, take a little water, add double the jaggery (for example, ¼ cup water and ½ cup of jaggery), and bring it to a boil to form a thick consistency. Add in the cardamom powder and mix well. Test it by putting a small drop in a small bowl of cold water; it should solidify immediately.
3. Remove from heat and add in the peanuts and sesame seeds. Mix well. The jaggery consistency should be thicker than the peanuts-and-sesame mixture.
4. Grease a separate plate with ghee and put the combined mixture into the plate, making it smooth with a spatula. Cut into 1" × 1" pieces while warm and allow the brittle to cool and solidify.

Baked Apple

Good for doshas: Vata and Pitta
Serving size: 1

Ingredients:
1 red apple
5 walnuts
1 teaspoon butter
¼ teaspoon brown sugar or maple syrup
⅛ teaspoon cinnamon powder
⅛ cup oats
A pinch of salt

Method:
1. Cut the red apple into long pieces. Crush the walnuts into small pieces.
2. Preheat the oven to 350 degrees Fahrenheit.
3. Put apple pieces, butter, brown sugar, salt, walnuts, and cinnamon powder in a saucepan. Cook for 10 minutes.
4. Transfer the above mixture into an ovenproof dish and bake for 25 minutes. Remove from the oven, drizzle the oats on the top, and bake for another 5–10 minutes until light brown.
5. Remove and enjoy warm.

Chapter 14
Meal Plans by Dosha

(Please note that the meal plans provided below are simply a guideline of how the plans should be designed per constitution, taking into consideration heat [summer] and cold [winter]. The meal plans have been designed in accordance with the suggested serving size of "1" as shown in chapter 11, "Food Charts and Quantification," and in the above recipes. These meal plans have been created with guidance from an Ayurvedacharya.)

Vata

Meal plans for the summer:

Meal	Plan 1	Plan 2
Breakfast	Grits / cream of wheat with ½ cup almond milk	One omelet made with green peppers, onions, tomatoes, spinach, and ginger
Snack	Pineapple or mango	Banana and sesame seeds
Lunch	Grilled fish and broccoli with buttered vegetable	Saffron basmati rice with sautéed mixed vegetables (carrots, peas, snow peas, and zucchini)
Snack	2 pieces (1" × 1" size) peanut brittle / chikki	Mixed nuts and raisins, cranberries, hazelnuts, walnuts, and macadamia nuts
Dinner	Chicken curry with brown rice	Moong and spinach dal

Meal plans for the winter:

Meal	Plan 1	Plan 2
Breakfast	Oatmeal cooked with cinnamon, walnuts, and ½ cup almond milk	Multigrain pancake with cardamom-saffron milk
Snack	Dry fruit smoothie	Baked apple
Lunch	Baked sweet potato with sautéed spinach, roasted mushrooms, and asparagus	Banana and fenugreek leaf vegetable with one roti
Snack	2 pieces (1" × 1" size) peanut brittle or chikki	Mixed nuts and raisins, prunes, and walnuts
Dinner	Whole moong dal with brown rice	Chicken curry and quinoa with carrots

Meal Plans by Dosha

Pitta

Meal plans for the summer:

Meal	Plan 1	Plan 2
Breakfast	2 egg whites and 1 piece of multigrain toast with herbal tea	Muesli and bran cereal with ½ cup almond or skim milk
Snack	Greek yogurt with a couple of walnuts	Fresh strawberries and raspberries
Lunch	Garden salad with grilled chicken	Banana and fenugreek leaf vegetable with one roti and 8-ounce glass of mint lassi
Snack	Pear or watermelon slice and an 8-ounce glass of coconut water	Carrots and cucumber with hummus
Dinner	Brown rice khicchadi with chicken curry	Moong and spinach dal with leek-flavored quinoa

Meal plans for the winter:

Meal	Plan 1	Plan 2
Breakfast	Oatmeal cooked with walnuts with ½ cup skim milk	Gram flour pancake with mango pickle and herbal tea
Snack	Soaked almonds and figs	Pomegranates or gooseberries
Lunch	Steamed cauliflower, carrots, and broccoli with garlic-flavored potatoes	Adzuki beans with couscous and carrots
Snack	Grapes and pumpkin seeds	Apple and sunflower seeds
Dinner	Moong and spinach dal	Roasted butternut squash soup

Kapha

Meal plans for the summer:

Meal	Plan 1	Plan 2
Breakfast	Cooked millet and herbal tea with ½ teaspoon honey	2 egg whites and a piece of rye toast with herbal tea
Snack	Strawberries and blueberries	Raspberries or a peach
Lunch	Chicken salad and a side of cooked beets	Corn khicchadi and a side of cooked radish
Snack	Cashews and pumpkin seeds	Kale chips
Dinner	Yellow dal with fenugreek leaves	Adzuki beans and cumin quinoa

Meal plans for the winter:

Meal	Plan 1	Plan 2
Breakfast	Oatmeal with ½ cup of almond milk	Moong dal pancake (adai)
Snack	Raspberries and pecans	Pumpkin seeds
Lunch	Vegetable and barley soup	Chicken curry with cumin quinoa
Snack	Kale chips	Green tea and cashews
Dinner	Bajra rotla and whole moong dal	Carrot and broccoli soup with rye toast

Chapter 15
Moong Soup—Detox Therapy

(Note: Please consult an Ayurvedacharya or medical doctor before doing this diet if you have any specific medical needs or chronic illness or are pregnant.)

The moong soup is used as part of a detox therapy to be incorporated after you have eaten some vegetarian meals. However, this can be used if one is trying to lose weight, since it aids in losing about 5 pounds in about fifteen days. It cleanses the body, removing any undigested toxins, or *Ama*, with a special focus on the liver and the gallbladder. It also helps with the issue of water retention and sharpens the digestive fire, which can become dull due to toxin accumulation.

It is suggested to have 1 teaspoon of ghee in hot water or ¼ teaspoon of castor oil in a cup of warm chamomile tea on a daily basis for three days prior to starting the therapy. You can consume this soup every three to four hours for all meals. If you feel very weak or tired, you can incorporate a little brown rice with the soup. In Ayurveda, it is prescribed to make a fresh pot of the soup each day, rather than reheat leftover soup. While doing this detox therapy, you may find it beneficial to incorporate walking, yoga, Pranayama breathing techniques, and a daily meditation practice for twenty to thirty minutes. If you cannot do all of these, even choosing one or two practices daily will be helpful.

Moong Soup Recipe

(The quantity has been provided for one meal portion. Please increase in proportion for total number of meals for the day.)

Ingredients:
¼ cup green moong beans
½ teaspoon ghee
½ teaspoon cumin seeds
5–8 small pieces of zucchini or bottle gourd
¼ inch fresh ginger, chopped finely
A pinch of hing or asafoetida
¼ teaspoon turmeric powder
1½ cups of water
Salt to taste
Lemon juice to taste

Method:
1. Wash the moong beans and soak for 4 hours before cooking.
2. Heat ghee in a pot; add the cumin seeds, zucchini or bottle gourd, fresh ginger, and pinch of asafoetida (or hing), then sauté.
3. Add in the soaked moong beans and turmeric powder, then sauté.
4. Add the water and cook until the beans are soft. You can also use a pressure cooker to cook the beans. It should not take more than 8 to 10 minutes once the pressure cooker is hot.
5. Once cooked, add the salt and lemon juice and serve hot.

Chapter 16
Panchakarma-Related Therapies

(Please consult your doctor/Ayurvedacharya before undertaking the Panchakarma therapies, to take into consideration any individual or specific medical conditions.)

Panchakarma is a five-therapy process that is used for detoxifying the body, rejuvenating the *Ojas* or immunity, and restoring a natural, healthy balance in mind and body. The word *Panchakarma* means five (*pancha*) actions (*karma*). Indigestion, stress, and negative emotions lead to the accumulation of toxins or *Ama* in the body, which affect all the organs and dull the digestive fire. The Panchakarma therapies are a method to remove the accumulated toxins in the body, cleanse and rejuvenate the entire system, and open up the energy channels, resulting in overall well-being. The actual Panchakarma therapies are *Vamana* (emesis), *Virechana* (purgation), *Basti* (medicinal enema), *Nasya* (nasal administration), and *Raktamoshana* (blood detoxification).

Some of these and other techniques used in Panchakarma include the following:

Abhayanga—where herbal oils are massaged into the entire body from head to toe to loosen up the toxins from the tissue layers and increase circulation, resulting in calmer nerves, joint lubrication, increased stamina, softer skin, and improved sleep. The oil can be warmed, applied to the body, and left to be absorbed by the skin. Massage using your fingers. Apply more oil to the nerve endings, such as the soles of the feet, fingers, and palms of the hands. On the rounder parts of the body, such as your head and joints, do the massage in a circular motion. After this has been completed, relax for about fifteen minutes, so that the oil is entirely absorbed and the nerves become calm. You can take a warm bath at the end of the massage process.

Shirodhara—the use of warm herbal oil in a gentle stream over your forehead. This process is beneficial in removing stress and anxiety, relaxing the nerves, improving memory, enhancing hearing and vision, nourishing the scalp, and calming the mind, body, and spirit.

Nasya—placing herbal oil drops in the nasal passages, followed by a gentle facial massage, including the neck and shoulders. This procedure prevents early graying of the hair or loss of hair and alleviates pain caused by sinusitis, spondylitis, frozen shoulder, and headaches. In addition, it sharpens the sense organs, improves the skin, and helps prevent wrinkles.

Swedana—this involves a therapeutic application of heat to the different parts of the body in order to melt the toxins in the body and release them as sweat through the skin pores. This improves circulation, enhances skin elasticity, reduces muscle pains, and removes stiffness from the joints.

Basti—the use of herbal oil and other decoctions as enemas to remove toxins, especially from the colon. This procedure can help cure sexual disorders, constipation, hyperacidity, chronic pain, fatigue, and hemorrhoids, resulting in the rejuvenation of the body. Basti is usually not advised for people with issues such as diarrhea, shortness of breath, and anemia.

Once the Panchakarma detox process therapies have been completed, the Ayurvedacharya or Ayurvedic Wellness coach will recommend certain foods and herbs to strengthen and nourish the body, resulting in a strong digestive fire, improved immunity, and longevity. In addition to foods and herbs, regular Pranayama and meditation are also encouraged.

It is a good idea to follow the detox process with a regular spiritual practice. A morning gratitude prayer is a wonderful way to raise a positive energy internally, which will accompany you through the day's activities. In addition to gratitude, you are encouraged to do fifteen to thirty minutes of meditation to calm the nerves, quiet the mind, and become more open to higher guidance.

Chapter 17
Stress Reduction and Pranayama

Stress is anything that is detrimental to our well-being. If stress or pressure feels overwhelming and affects our physical and mental health, then the overall effect is negative, which can lead to illness, weight gain, and depression. Stress has become the fastest-spreading epidemic of the modern age—the times that we live in today. The pace of life has increased along with socioeconomic and political changes, higher cost of living, and various catastrophes each year. The external conditions, in addition to personal, individual situations, become overwhelming for a number of people.

Some of the symptoms of stress include:
- hypertension
- headaches
- pressure in the chest area and shallow, rapid breathing
- digestion slowing down and immunity being impaired
- muscles becoming tense
- normal sleep patterns being disturbed
- chest and back pain
- nail-biting
- stomach upsets
- fainting spells
- anger
- anxiety and burnout
- depression
- irritability
- exhaustion
- food cravings, which can lead to bingeing and weight gain

- relationship problems and social withdrawal
- drug and alcohol use

Stress can be caused by a number of reasons:
- financial pressures
- family problems
- relationship issues
- job problems and unemployment
- perceived lack of time
- bereavement
- miscarriage or abortion
- weight gain

In order to combat stress, there have been many recommendations made by professionals, including Ayurvedic specialists, such as exercise, deep breathing for stress relief, a healthful and balanced diet of fruits and vegetables, massage, yoga, support groups where people can comfortably discuss issues, or talking to a close friend or family member for encouragement and support.

The benefits of reducing stress are evident when you have more energy during the day, a restful sleep at night, and more vitality. You will find that negative emotions such as irritability, anger, frustration will diminish; and positive feelings of love, compassion, kindness, both for yourself and others, will increase. There will be more interest and joy in experiencing life to the fullest and in flowing with the Universe rather than struggling or going against the natural flow. If you are restricted by time constraints and cannot undertake all of the above, take baby steps by first changing your diet to include more natural foods. This way you will not feel overwhelmed by all the changes that you wish to make but will be able to enjoy the transition, step by step, and will be more determined to reach your ultimate goal.

Exercise is a wonderful way to reduce stress, remove toxins, and increase the flow of *Prana* in the body. In Ayurveda, exercise is recommended to increase energy, vitality, and mind-body coordination. Exercises can be delineated by dosha type:

> **Vata:** have bursts of energy and can get tired easily. Yoga is recommended for balance and grounding. The other exercises that are good for Vata individuals are walking and dancing. Cross-training and elliptical

machines are preferable to treadmills in the gym for Vata.

Pitta: include challenging sports such as mountain climbing, hiking, tennis, bicycling, and roller-blading. Water sports, especially swimming, are beneficial to Pitta, since these aid in having a cooling effect.

Kapha: have great strength and endurance, which allows them to take up exercises such as long-distance running, cycling, aerobics, and rowing. The main issue faced by Kapha individuals is that they are not generally inclined to an exercise routine and may prefer to start with a daily brisk walk.

It is true that not everyone can afford regular yoga classes and massages, but there are two vital practices that Ayurveda advises to reduce stress that are free, which are:

- meditation and spending high-quality time alone.
- Pranayama or breathing exercises.

So, what is meditation?

Meditation is a method to control or self-regulate the mind, bringing it to a place of single-pointed concentration to connect with one's higher self, consciousness, or what is also referred to as the *I AM* or the soul. It can be done by anyone, but it requires some practice, dedication, and commitment. Over time, it allows you to come into harmony and be synchronized with the universal laws to manifest the things you want in life. The effects have been sometimes described as *magic*!

In the age of technology, we have become accustomed to being bombarded with information from all kinds of media—books, television, and the internet. This has increased our logical, analytical, and rational mindsets, but in the bargain, we have lost our intrinsic connection to something that is far more precious—our inner being. Meditation can bring you back to yourself. It stills the mental chatter, body tension, and emotional stress. It allows you to realign yourself with the universal flow, avoid struggling, and learn self-acceptance. This creates a sense of calm, increases love and compassion, causes a radical shift in your emotional state, resulting in peace of mind and joy.

To meditate, all you need is a quiet place and time; you can sit in any position that keeps the body in balance comfortably and provides the least resistance to the flow of energy between the Universe and yourself.

The most common way is to sit comfortably in a cross-legged position; take an object—such as an orange, or flower, or for some it might be a picture of God or a candle—place it in front of you and keep looking at it, focusing only on that object. Try to assimilate the color, shape, and size. Focus on the object to develop your self-concentration abilities. If other thoughts interfere, let them come and go, gently releasing them, and going back to focusing on the specific object in front of you. Initially, this may happen for only about five minutes, but with time and practice, your focus will increase, your mental chatter will cease, and your mind and breathing will start to regulate, allowing you to be more open to the energetic vibrations of the Universe and the *I AM*. Pressure, tension, and worry will dissipate with each slow and deep breath, in the rhythmic rise and fall of each inhalation and exhalation.

Pranayama is the breathing method that has been espoused in the *Yoga Sutras of Patanjali*. *Prana* means life force and *yama* means control. Conscious breathing reduces stress and relaxes the individual. Pranayama is a breathing practice where every breath must be gentle, relaxing, invigorating, and not intense in nature.

Alternate-nostril breathing (*Nadi-Shodhan*) is the most common breathing exercise for stress relief.

- Sit in a cross-legged position, curl the index and middle finger of the right hand, and, using the right ring finger, close the left nostril.
- Inhale through the right nostril and hold the breath for a few seconds.
- Close the right nostril with the thumb, release the ring finger on the left nostril, and exhale slowly.
- Repeat the above process with the left nostril.
- Repeat the entire breathing exercise ten to fifteen times.

Breathing through the right nostril makes one more energetic, active, assertive, and generally in control. It has a positive effect on digestion and on daily performance. In the above practice, when one breathes through the left nostril, it makes one more spiritual, contemplative, and relaxed. The Nadi-Shodhan exercise as a whole balances you as you move further into the meditative process. If you have trouble shifting your breathing pattern to a slower pace for meditation, exhale by bringing in the abdomen completely, then inhale via both your nostrils and hold. This will force the breath to slow down and find a rhythm more suitable to you.

There are times when we are upset by inner turmoil or external circumstances, leading to frustration. One of the exercises to withdraw completely and get in tune with your *I AM* is described below:

- Sit on a chair or cross-legged on the floor, with the spine straight. Exhale and come to a relaxed pose.
- Using all the fingers of the hand on each side of the face, cover the ears (with the thumbs), eyes (with the index fingers), nose (with the middle fingers), and mouth (with the fourth and little fingers).
- Focus on an object in your mind.
- Breathe in deeply, bringing the stomach in completely.
- Remove the middle finger from the left nostril and exhale deeply, pushing the stomach out. Put the finger back on the left nostril and, removing the finger from the right nostril, inhale deeply, bringing the stomach completely in.
- Repeat the process multiple times, alternating the nostrils. Continue to keep the focus on the object in your mind.
- Slowly the mind will relax and finally stop; with continued practice, it also might be possible to see your own life-light internally.

There are some specific Pranayama exercises for each dosha. One of the best breathing exercises both for Pitta and Vata doshas is *Shitali*, since it has a cooling effect and is relaxing for the nervous system. Shitali breathing is described below:

- Sit in a cross-legged position.
- Roll the tongue, curling the sides in to form a longitudinal cylinder/tube, or make an *O* shape with the lips.
- Stick the tongue out of the mouth.
- Inhale through the tube of the mouth and exhale through the nose.
- Repeat ten to fifteen times to get a relaxed, cooling effect.

The *breath of fire* or *Kapalbhati* breathing exercise is beneficial for Kapha dosha:

- Inhale and exhale through the nose, making a quick, snorting sound while drawing the belly button / abdomen in powerfully, like a *pumping* action.
- Repeat about ten to fifteen times for each round.
- It is advocated to do only seven to ten rounds of this at a time.

Both meditation and Pranayama as a regular daily practice will help reduce stress, bring joy, and connect the individual to the Universe—the connection between *Atma* (individual soul) and *Paramatma* (God or Higher Self).

Chapter 18
The Art of Mindfulness

Mindfulness is to *just be* in the present moment. It is the attentive awareness of the reality of things. It is the practice of *doing less* and gaining more, because by being in the moment with complete alertness, you are connecting with the power and energy of the universal forces to get answers that you need without much external effort, along with sustenance at a molecular level too. By not being in the moment, you lose the valuable gift of being able to understand the bigger picture.

The activities of meditation and Pranayama are two ways of performing mindfulness. However, in practical day-to-day living, there are many other ways to be mindful. If you are drinking a cup of tea, for example, do just that in total absorption, without multitasking. You'll find that the cup of tea will taste better. Another way is by listening to music. Music is a universal language, crossing all boundaries and binding people together. When you are listening to music, become aware of each sound and vibration of the music being played in the current moment.

One of the best spiritual exercises that can support you in your daily life is when you are both the *observer* and the *observed*. It is when you are aware, nonjudgmental, and mindfully examine your thoughts and actions, that you gain insight on how to modify your behavior patterns. You become the external observer who watches the actions of the *subject*—yourself—to allow a conscious correction of your thoughts or actions in any instance, resulting in positivity. Mindfulness increases awareness in your thoughts, actions, reactions, and feelings.

The above concept has been taken from the ancient Hindu scriptures, in which there is a story of two birds—one (the observer) is sitting still and silent on the top branch, and the other (the subject being observed) is on the bottom branch of a tree, hopping from one branch to another, chirping constantly. The bird at the top objectively watches the movements and actions of the bird on the bottom. It should be noted, however, that in essence, the two birds are really one and the same. It is only when you are mindful, a silent witness, and aware of your actions on a subconscious level that you can create new, benevolent, and more productive neurological patterns in your brain, resulting in happiness.

If we consider this from the viewpoint of food and health, it is natural to have cravings, even if you have healthful eating habits. Mindfulness while eating will help satisfy the cravings, without a feeling of deprivation, or emotional binging. It is through mindfulness that you come to understand that *it is really the mind that needs to be put on a diet* to remove any self-sabotaging thoughts about your body and overall well-being.

Chapter 19
Understanding Chakra Energy

Everything in the Universe emits energy and has a radiation pattern. The human energy field, or *aura*, is the electromagnetic field that surrounds or emits from the human body. It has the ability to nourish each cell in the body and is supplied energy by the *Chakras* or *vortexes*. It is essential that these Chakras remain unblocked to experience harmony and ease in the mental, physical, and emotional bodies. By removing any blocks, awareness levels are raised, which in turn promotes spiritual growth, and the ultimate connection between *Atma* and *Paramatma*.

There are a number of subtle energy cycles within the body, but there are seven main Chakras that are located along the central channel (*Sushumna*), which appear in the form of petal formations. Here is an overview of the seven main Chakras and an understanding of your emotional and physical states at any point of time:

Mooldhara (Root) Chakra:
Location: base of the spine.
Intrinsic benefit: to find one's purpose in daily living.
Physical effect of blocked Chakra: exhaustion, obesity, sciatica, knee pain, weaker immunity, and constipation.
Emotional effect of blocked Chakra: insecurity, depression, anger, and commitment issues.

Swadhisthana (Sacral) Chakra:
Location: above the pubic bone and below the navel, covering the genitals
Intrinsic benefit: increases creativity and joy of life.
Physical effect of blocked Chakra: sexual libido issues, poor digestion, hormonal imbalance, urinary tract issues, and skin-related ailments.
Emotional effect of blocked Chakra: shyness, irritability, low creativity, addictions, intimacy, rejection, betrayal, and abandonment issues.

Manipura (Solar Plexus) Chakra:

Location: upper abdomen.

Intrinsic benefit: increases personal power, will, and responsibility of one's own life and achievements.

Physical effect of blocked Chakra: poor digestion, weight problems, liver issues, diabetes, intestinal tumors, and colon issues.

Emotional effect of blocked Chakra: distrust, seeks others' approval, image issues, feels like he/she is not good enough, judgmental, self-critical, and demanding.

Anhata (Heart) Chakra:

Location: center of the chest.

Intrinsic benefit: trust and love in the Universe.

Physical effect of blocked Chakra: heart ailments, back and shoulder aches, asthma, breathing and lung-related disorders.

Emotional effect of blocked Chakra: fear, jealousy, hopelessness, bitterness, loneliness, anxiousness, lack of self-love, self-esteem issues, and constant distress.

Vishuddha (Throat) Chakra:

Location: in the throat region, near the spine.

Intrinsic benefit: listening to and following one's intuition.

Physical effect of blocked Chakra: throat disorders, thyroid dysfunction, ear infection, sinus issues, and laryngitis.

Emotional effect of blocked Chakra: communication issues, unable to open up emotionally, lack of creativity, self-expression issues, and being self-critical.

Ajna (Brow) Chakra:

Location: center of the forehead.

Intrinsic benefit: spiritual insight and search for Universal Truth.

Physical effect of blocked Chakra: weak eyesight, blurred vision, headaches, migraines, and nightmares.

Emotional effect of blocked Chakra: fear of truth, lack of spiritual perception,

concentration issues, stubbornness, moodiness, and being opinionated.
Sahasrara (Crown) Chakra:
Location: on the crown of the head beneath the fontanelle.
Intrinsic benefit: spiritual realization and enlightenment.
Physical effect of blocked Chakra: sensitivity to light and sound.
Emotional effect of blocked Chakra: lack of motivation or purpose, no life direction, rigidity in thinking, and a feeling of constant restriction.

The table illustrates examples of foods that are beneficial for balancing and stimulate the Chakras listed below:

Chakra	Foods to Balance and Stimulate
Root	Apple, radish, beetroot, carrots, potato, yam, sweet potato, radish, onions, strawberries
Sacral	Pumpkin, nuts, melon, mango, orange, tangerine, honey
Solar plexus	Whole grains, corn, yellow pepper, banana, pineapple
Heart	Lettuce, kale, broccoli, green beans, bean sprouts, lentils
Throat	Barley, mushroom, blueberries, blackberries, dragon fruit
Third eye	Eggplant, purple lettuce, grapes, black currants, prunes
Crown	No specific foods—advice is to fast and detox mentally and physically

Chapter 20
Yoga Asanas to Improve *Agni*

Surya namaskar:

This is a set of twelve postures that improves the alignment of the spine, strengthens the muscles, and dissolves inches from the waist, bringing a complete sense of contentment. The postures are beneficial in increasing the digestive and metabolic fire in the gastrointestinal tract. The entire practice does not take more than twenty minutes (about six to ten repetitions) to complete and is a great way to start the day.

In addition, there are certain yoga postures that can be practiced to improve your digestion. The poses are:

- Backward Bend / Sphinx—*Salamba Bhujangasana*
- Boat—*Navasana*
- Bow—*Dhanurasana*
- Bridge—*Setu Bandha Sarvangasana*
- Camel—*Ustrasana*
- Cat and Cow—*Marjariasana*
- Child's Pose—*Balasana*
- Cobra—*Bhujangasana*
- Corpse—*Sarvasana*
- Downward-Facing Dog—*Adho Mukha Svanasana*
- Forward Bend—*Uttanasana*
- Hero—*Virasana*
- Plow—*Halasana*
- Spinal Twist—*Supta Matsyendrasana*
- Triangle—*Trikonasana*
- Upward-Facing Dog—*Urdhva Mukha Svanasana*
- Wind Release—*Pavanmuktasana*

Chapter 21
Common Ailments and the Suggested Ayurvedic Remedies

(Please note that all recommendations have been made by an Ayurvedacharya or Ayurvedic doctor. The details regarding the herbs have been provided for informational purpose, and it is preferable to initially use diet and lifestyle changes to heal. For any prolonged ailment or a specific dosage, including advice on herbs to suit your individual constitution/dosha, please consult an Ayurvedic doctor or Ayurvedacharya before ingesting any herbs.)

The Oxford dictionary has described the word *disease* as *a disorder of structure or function in a human, especially one that produces specific signs or symptoms or that affects a specific location and is not simply a direct result of physical injury.*[1] The origin of the word is from Middle English, in which *disease* actually means *lack of ease* or *inconvenience*.

According to the ancient science of Ayurveda, all disease starts when you are not living in harmony with nature. If anything negative is absorbed through the five senses, it weakens the body and the muscles become tense, affecting the vertebrae and the connected nerves, which causes a complete disruption in the energy flow and results in *Ama*. It is believed in Ayurveda that *Ama* is the root of all diseases.

Ama, as we have learned, is the accumulated, undigested matter in our gastro-intestinal tract that results in a weak digestive system and compromised immunity. The Ayurvedacharya takes into consideration the individual internal flow or your unique constitution to prescribe the remedies. However, in general, lowering stress and generating empowering thoughts are part of the individual healing process.

The list below highlights some common ailments and diseases:

Acne

Symptoms: Skin disorder that causes the formation of pimples or lesions on the face, chest, or back.

Causes: It is caused by an overproduction of sebum, and, metaphysically, it is considered to be due to a lack of self-love or not accepting oneself.

Ayurvedic connotation: Acne is an imbalance of Pitta and is onset at the time of puberty.

Suggested Remedies:

Diet: A cooling and bland alkaline diet is advised. The foods include dark-green leafy vegetables, whole grains, sweet fruits (except citrus fruits), and other vegetables (except tomatoes). Coriander-cumin-fennel tea is also prescribed, along with plenty of water (preferably at room temperature).

Lifestyle: Avoid late nights, alcohol, caffeine, cigarettes, and other stimulants. Regular exercise, proper care for skin or personal hygiene, and adequate sleep are suggested. If you are constipated, please refer to the remedy under this ailment in the list below.

Yoga: Postures that reduce stress and improve blood circulation—Downward-Facing Dog and Shoulder Stand.

Pranayama: Shitali, Kapalbhati, and Anuloma-Viloma (alternate-nostril breathing).

Herbs: Triphala, Aloe Vera juice, and Neem (disinfectant).

Bronchitis

Symptoms: Fever, chills, muscle aches, nasal congestion, and sore throat, with a cough being the most common symptom. The cough can be dry or may produce phlegm. Forceful coughing could cause pain in the chest and abdominal muscles, along with wheezing and shortness of breath.

Causes: It is caused by an upper respiratory infection, such as a cold or sinus infection; metaphysically, it may be due to an inflamed family environment.

Ayurvedic connotation: Kapha and Vata related congestion disease.

Suggested Remedies:

Diet: Food and herbal teas with warming spices such as black pepper, ginger, basil, cinnamon, and turmeric help open and cleanse the respiratory channel. It is suggested to have warm, cooked foods during the fall, winter, and spring seasons. Avoid raw and frozen foods, especially those containing cheese, yogurt, and gluten.

Lifestyle: Gentle nasal wash (neti pots).

Yoga: Corpse, Shoulder Lift, Half-Spinal Twist, and Wind-Relieving poses.

Pranayama: Anuloma-Viloma (alternate-nostril breathing).

Herbs: Trikatu tablets, Licorice, and Honey.

Cholesterol (LDL: Low-Density Lipoprotein)

Symptoms: LDL carries more fat and less protein from the liver to other parts of the body, resulting in the clogging of the arteries, and can lead to serious problems such as heart attack and stroke.

Causes: The common causes are foods with saturated fat or transfat, age, inactivity, genetics, and hypothyroidism. Metaphysically, it is the obstruction of the channels of joy.

Ayurvedic connotation: Improper processing of lipids and imbalanced fat metabolism in the body. Toxin-infused fat deposits choke up the internal channels in the body, creating blood-circulation issues.

Suggested Remedies:

Diet: Increase the use of ginger, garlic, onion, and cayenne pepper in your food. It is suggested to eat more green leafy vegetables and use healthful oils such as olive oil and ghee. Avoid fried foods and foods with saturated fats and transfat.

Lifestyle: Daily exercise (at least for thirty minutes), yoga, and Pranayama. Eat at regular intervals (only when hungry) and drink hot water continually throughout the day.

Yoga: Surya Namaskar (the twelve-pose routine) and Corpse pose.

Pranayama: Anuloma-Viloma and Kapalbhati.

Herbs: Guggul compounds *(please consult with an Ayurvedacharya for more information).*

Chronic Fatigue

Symptoms: Exhaustion that has lasted for six months or more and does not improve with rest. It can lead to fever, sore throat, muscle pain, headaches, and feeling sick after exercising. It can be related to iron and calcium deficiencies in the body. In Pitta individuals especially, it can cause acidic indigestion, leading to high blood pressure, irritation, and joint pain.

Causes: Smoking, malnutrition (micronutrient deficiency), viral infection, environmental reasons, diabetes, and emotional events (depression). Metaphysically, it is a doorway to different forms of release and access to new outlooks.

Ayurvedic connotation: It is considered to be a blockage in the physical, emotional, and subtle pathways of the mind and body. It is caused by a low metabolic fire.

Suggested Remedies:

Diet: Lightly roasted whole grains, sprouts, green leafy vegetables, some nuts (almonds and walnuts), seeds (sesame and sunflower), and fruits such as berries and cherries (which are high in antioxidants) should be eaten. Avoid red meat, gluten, tofu, processed foods, and baked goods. Drink hot water continually during the day, along with cumin tea.

Lifestyle: Daily exercise, yoga, walking, and swimming are advocated along with a regular *Dinacharya*, or daily routine.

Yoga: Child's Pose, Bridge, Head-to-Knee Forward-Bend, and Legs-Up-the-Wall poses.

Pranayama: Kapalabhati, Shitali, Anuloma-Viloma, Brahmari, and Ujjayi.

Herbs: Trikatu, Ashwagandha, and Licorice.

Constipation

Symptoms: When one is having a bowel movement less than three times a week, accompanied by difficulty or pain while passing stools.

Causes: The common causes are a low-fiber diet, lack of physical activity, insufficient water consumption, stress, underactive thyroid, and use of certain medications. Metaphysically, it is the refusal to release old ideas.

Ayurvedic connotation: Vata imbalance due to irregular lifestyle and eating habits. Dehydration is a common cause. Too much travel can aggravate this imbalance.

Suggested Remedies:

Diet: Eat more high-fiber, freshly cooked foods—green leafy vegetables, natural oats, brown rice—and drink more hot water. It is suggested to use digestive spices such as fennel, ginger, and cumin.

Lifestyle: Daily exercise is essential, along with eating at regular intervals (only when hungry).

Yoga: Cobra, Plow, Twist, Hero, Wind-Relieving, Head-to-Knee Forward-Bend, Back-Spine Stretching, and Corpse poses.

Pranayama: Kapalabhati and Anuloma-Viloma.

Herbs: Castor oil, Triphala, and Haritaki.

Diabetes

Symptoms: Fatigue, stress, unexplained weight loss, excessive thirst, increased urination, and a higher intake of food. It can lead to yeast infection, urinary tract infection, irritability, agitation, and extreme lethargy.

Causes: Genetics (diabetes has strong genetic links), a high-fat diet, obesity, sedentary lifestyle, high alcohol intake, aging, and ethnicity. Metaphysically, it is due to the lack of sweetness in life and longing for what could have been.

Ayurvedic connotation: It is known to be caused due to a Kapha aggravated dosha, but in some cases can also be a Pitta related disease.

Suggested Remedies:

Diet: Bitter gourd (*karela*) is specifically prescribed, as well as green leafy vegetables, lentils, legumes, whole grains (barley, millet, quinoa, and oats), turmeric, fenugreek, cinnamon, and cumin. Avoid gluten and starchy tuberous vegetables (sweet potato and yam). Buttermilk in the summer is recommended.

Lifestyle: Increase the exercise routine, especially walking (minimum thirty to forty-five minutes daily).

Yoga: Downward-Facing Dog, Triangle, Hero, Fish, Corpse, Half-Lord of the Fishes, and Twist poses.

Pranayama: Kapalabhati and Anuloma-Viloma.

Herbs: Gudmar, Amalaki, and Guggul compounds *(please consult with an Ayurvedacharya for more information).*

Eczema

Symptoms: Eczema is a type of skin inflammation. Intense itching is the main symptom, and it can result in a dry, reddened, and scaly skin. The other symptoms include cracked or broken skin; inflamed areas in the skin can develop blisters or small, raised bumps.

Causes: It is considered to be a genetic condition that can be aggravated by environmental factors, exposure to certain substances/materials, hormone fluctuations, and stress. It can also be caused by certain dietary products such as milk, wheat, peanuts, and eggs. Metaphysically, it is due to feeling unworthy or inadequate.

Ayurvedic connotation: Impurities from blood and lymph, when saturated in the form of *Ama* (toxins), get expelled from the skin pores and create the above symptoms due to their irritant nature. Ama is also created when Pitta is out of balance in the body, mind, *Agni*, and hormones, causing the clogging of the skin surface.

Suggested Remedies:

Diet: Alkaline, cooling, natural foods such as leafy green vegetables and sprouts. Fruits rich in antioxidants are preferable. The use of turmeric while cooking the vegetables is suggested.

Lifestyle: Meditation is very beneficial, since it calms the mind and body.

Yoga: Plough, Child, Cobra, Corpse, Shoulder Stand, and Surya Namaskar poses.

Pranayama: Kapalabhati, Anuloma-Viloma, and Nadi-Shodhan.

Herbs: Neem, Aloe Vera, Manjistha, and Triphala.

Food Allergies

Symptoms: An allergic reaction to a food item can be uncomfortable, frightening, or even life-threatening. The symptoms usually develop within a few minutes to two hours after eating the "offending" food item. It can result in tingling in the mouth; itching; eczema; swelling of the lips, tongue, or face; trouble breathing; wheezing; dizziness; abdominal pain; nausea; diarrhea; and even fainting.

Causes: The body's immune system mistakenly identifies a food as harmful. It can be triggered by certain proteins in food items such as shellfish, peanuts, walnuts, pecans, eggs, and milk. Metaphysically, it is dealing with repressed emotions or beliefs and a need to raise self-love.

Ayurvedic connotation: The food is altered genetically or chemically in a form that is not digested by the body and results in an allergy. In addition, emotional disturbance can cause a negative impact on the mind and body, resulting in allergies.

Suggested Remedies:

Diet: Organic and fresh foods, especially green vegetables and fruits rich in antioxidants. It is suggested to avoid any artificial or processed foods, especially those foods that are the cause of the allergy (milk, nuts, etc.), until the body is brought into balance. The use of turmeric is good for cleansing the blood and pacifying the Pitta constitution.

Lifestyle: Meditation is suggested along with a *Chakra evaluation* for an understanding of deep-rooted fears. This will assist in increasing willpower and self-confidence. *(A Chakra evaluation can be done by an Ayurvedic Holistic Health practitioner, spiritual healer, or, in some cases, an Ayurvedacharya.)*

Yoga: Surya Namaskar, Wind-Relieving, Triangle, Mountain, Fish, Plow, Serpent, and Hare poses.

Pranayama: Shitali, Nadi-Shodhan, and Seethkari.

Herbs: Guduchi, Amalaki, Sandalwood, and Brahmi.

Headache

Symptoms: Pain or discomfort in the head, scalp, and neck.

Causes: Stress, depression, anxiety, head injury, and holding the head or neck in an abnormal position. Metaphysically, it is not accepting what is going on, along with self-criticism.

Ayurvedic connotation: The following unstable factors lead to headaches: Vata imbalance causes dehydration, dry sinuses, insomnia, constipation, and stressful thinking. Pitta imbalance caused by excessive alcohol, spicy food, work pressure, competition, late nights. Kapha imbalance caused due to exposure to cold, wind, rain; which results in sinus congestion and building up of mucus and phlegm leading to pressure. In addition to these, headaches can be caused by hypoglycemia, hypertension, hunger, acidity, and other neurological issues.

Suggested Remedies:

Diet: Freshly cooked nonacidic food, green leafy vegetables, root vegetables, fruits, milk, and nuts (almonds, walnuts). Fennel, coriander, and ginger are beneficial. It is counseled to use ghee while cooking your food.

Lifestyle: Follow a proper Dinacharya routine. A head massage with coconut or *Brahmi* oil is beneficial.

Yoga: Cat, Half-Twist, Mountain, and Chest-Opening poses.

Pranayama: Bhastrika and Kapalabhati.

Herbs: Amalaki.

Common Ailments and the Suggested Ayurvedic Remedies

Insomnia

Symptoms: A sleep disorder with a difficulty in falling or staying asleep (or both). It also involves waking up during the night and having a problem going back to sleep, or waking up too early in the morning and being tired upon waking up. This results in sleepiness during the day, irritability, general tiredness, and lack of concentration.

Causes: Life stress, emotional or physical discomfort, illness, environmental factors, and certain medications. Metaphysically, it is not having the ability to trust life due to stress and fear.

Ayurvedic connotation: It is a Vata imbalance caused by irregular sleep patterns, improper lifestyle, and use of stimulants (e.g., alcohol and caffeine).

Suggested Remedies:

Diet: Warm root vegetables, whole grains, dairy products, fruits such as banana, and chamomile tea. You are encouraged to use ghee while cooking your food.

Lifestyle: Daily meditation practice is essential; also yoga, Pranayama, and walking (thirty to forty-five minutes daily).

Yoga: Child's Pose, Forward Bend, Plow, Seated Forward-Bend, Spinal Twist, and Shoulder Stand poses.

Pranayama: Ujjayi.

Herbs: Brahmi oil or Coconut oil can be used for a foot and scalp massage.

Common Ailments and the Suggested Ayurvedic Remedies

Irregular Menstrual Cycle

Symptoms: Irregular periods are the first sign that a woman is approaching menopause, or, in younger women, it could be due to hormonal imbalances. Women experience irregular periods for three to ten years before the periods stop entirely. The symptoms are missed periods, painful cramps, abnormal duration, changes in the blood flow, and blood clots.

Causes: Fluctuating hormone levels for women between the ages of forty-five and fifty-five. It is also caused by certain health conditions such as irritable bowel syndrome (IBS), thyroid dysfunction, miscarriage, liver disease, cancer, diabetes, and eating disorders. In addition, lifestyle triggers such as overexercise, significant weight gain or loss, smoking, caffeine intake, excessive alcohol consumption, increased stress, and poor nutrition can cause an imbalance. Metaphysically, it is a rejection of one's femininity and a feeling of guilt.

Ayurvedic connotation: It is a Pitta and Vata imbalance. Pitta imbalance can create hormonal fluctuations and irregular bleeding patterns. Vata imbalance can cause delayed and scanty periods with pain or cramps. It is only when the Vata in the pelvic organ is redirected in the normal pathways (downward and outward flow), along with a hormonal balance for Pitta, that regular menstruation is established.

Suggested Remedies:

Diet: The Pitta imbalance should be counteracted by an increased intake of alkaline foods such as green leafy vegetables and fruits high in antioxidants. You are urged to have warm and cooked foods (not raw salads) to bring the Vata into balance. Spices such as asafoetida, fennel, sesame, fenugreek, cumin, ajwain, and jaggery can be used. Grape or carrot juice may be added to the diet.

Lifestyle: Meditation and Pranayama to reduce any stress that may be affecting the regular cycle. If you smoke or consume excessive alcohol or coffee, you are counseled to give up such habits.

Yoga: Cow, Head-to-Knee Forward-Bend, Cobra, Hero, Lion, and Cobbler poses.

Pranayama: Kapalabhati and Anuloma-Viloma.

Herbs: Aloe vera, Shatavari, and Dashamoola. The application of an oil (sesame or castor oil) patch on the navel is suggested *(please do a test on a small part of your skin before application to ensure that you are not allergic to the oil).*

Irritable Bowel Syndrome

Symptoms: A combination of abdominal discomfort and altered bowel habits. The symptoms are diarrhea or constipation, abdominal pain or cramps, and excessive gas.

Causes: Problem of bowel mobility, certain foods, medicines, and emotional stress. Metaphysically, it is feeling upset at the opposite sex.

Ayurvedic connotation: IBS is a result of a Pitta and Vata imbalance in one's agni, which causes a weak, uneven digestive fire and improper peristaltic activity, respectively. This indicates a need to improve the metabolic fire which can be done by following regular eating habits, small balanced meals, and warm water.

Suggested Remedies:

Diet: It is best to eat freshly cooked food and avoid leftovers. Foods such as root vegetables, cooked zucchini, pumpkin, apples, bananas, pears (all cooked), rice, and yogurt are beneficial. Avoid gluten-based foods and meat products. Spices such as cumin, carom seeds, black salt, garlic (cooked), nutmeg, ginger, fennel, fenugreek, and coriander/cilantro can be included while cooking.

Lifestyle: A proper daily routine, gentle yoga to improve the peristaltic activity, OM meditation, and Pranayama. It is advised to use more grounding, relaxing techniques for better assimilation and absorption of food.

Yoga: Corpse, Eagle, Wide-Angle Seated, Downward Dog, Headstand, Shoulder Stand, Half-Plow, Wind-Relieving, Bridge, and Surya Namaskar poses.

Pranayama: Kapalabhati and Nadi-Shodhan.

Herbs: Kutaj tablets.

Kidney Failure

Symptoms: Kidneys stop working and the waste products build up in the body. The main symptoms are swelling in the legs and feet, little or no urine when one goes to urinate, no appetite, nausea, anxiousness, restlessness, and pain in the back.

Causes: Reduced blood flow to the kidneys due to an injury, blood loss, or an infection; damage caused due to certain medications such as aspirin or ibuprofen; and kidney stones that stop the urine from flowing out of the kidneys. Metaphysically, it is due to criticism or shame.

Ayurvedic connotation: This is a Kapha imbalance upsetting the fluid circulation and metabolism in the body. It causes the stagnation of fluids [which contain a higher concentration of waste materials], bloating, overwhelms the lymphatic system, retains water in the area of extremities, and results in weight gain.

Suggested Remedies:

Diet: Foods that are astringent (that dry up the fluid)—green tea, roasted grains such as brown rice and millet, and raw vegetable juice. Cranberry or orange juice (with low sugar content) along with Aloe Vera is good for flushing. Citrus fruits such as oranges, grapefruit, or tangerines are suggested so long as the individual does not have a Pitta imbalance. Avoid cheese, gluten products, and white flour. Reduce dairy intake, especially any dairy with high fat and protein. Spices such as black pepper, fennel, coriander, cumin, turmeric, and cardamom are suggested.

Lifestyle: Daily exercise, eating on a regular schedule, and more fluid intake (water) to cleanse the lymphatic system and kidneys.

Yoga: Cobra, Twist, Pigeon, Back Bend, Head-to-Knee, and Half-Spinal Twist poses.

Pranayama: Anuloma-Viloma, Bhastrika, Brahmari, Nadi-Shodhan, and Kapalabhati.

Herbs: Triphala, Sandalwood, Punarnava, Guggul, and Dashamoola.

Kidney Stones

Symptoms: Kidney stones may not have symptoms (silent) or can have symptoms such as cramping pain in the lower back, groin, and abdomen, accompanied by nausea, fever, chills, or the appearance of blood in the urine.

Causes: It is caused when the normal balance of water, salt, minerals, and other substances found in the urine changes. The most common cause for this change is not drinking enough water. The other causes are heredity and medical conditions such as gout or Crohn's disease. Metaphysically, it is due to unresolved anger.

Ayurvedic connotation: Primarily a Kapha imbalance, but it is also aggravated by a Vata imbalance in the body.

Suggested Remedies:

Diet: Avoid processed or artificial foods such as sodas, coffee, white flour, and cheese. Increase more fluids such as water, cranberry juice, and citrus fruits to flush the kidneys. Spices such as cardamom, fenugreek, and cumin are suggested.

Lifestyle: Regular exercise and diet (*note*—it is essential to increase the intake of water).

Yoga: Bow, Wind-Relieving, Raised Feet, and Plow poses.

Pranayama: Anuloma-Viloma, Kapalabhati, and Brahmari.

Herbs: Triphala, Sandalwood, Punarnava, Guggul, and Dashamoola.

Common Ailments and the Suggested Ayurvedic Remedies

Memory Issues

Symptoms: Memory loss or unusual forgetfulness. One may not be able to remember new events, recall past events, or both.

Causes: Alcohol, drugs, not enough oxygen to the brain, aging, constant multitasking lifestyle, ADHD, cancer, tumor, certain medications, head trauma, depression, migraines, lack of sleep, stress, smoking, hormonal imbalances, and nutritional problems (nutrient deficiency). Metaphysically, it is not letting go of the past and living in the moment.

Ayurvedic connotation: Vata imbalance in the mind leads to short-term memory loss due to lack of concentration and not being present in the moment.

Suggested Remedies:

Diet: Organic fresh food and antioxidant fruits, ghee, garlic, white pumpkin, almonds, and walnuts.

Lifestyle: OM meditation, chanting mantras (repetition brings you to the present moment and helps increase concentration).

Yoga: Shoulder Stand, Tree, and Cobra poses. Focus is increased by holding the balancing poses for a longer time.

Pranayama: Bhastrika, Kapalabhati, and Brahmari.

Herbs: Brahmi, Gotukola, and Shankhapushpi.

Menstrual Symptoms and Menopause

Menopause symptoms: Natural menopause is a permanent ending of menstruation. Menopause is the point when it has been a year since a woman last had her menstrual period. The symptoms are hot flashes, skipped periods, insomnia, mood swings, fatigue, depression, irritability, headaches, vaginal dryness, bladder control problems, gas, dryness of the skin, lack of interest in sex, digestive disorders, weight gain, postmenopausal diabetes, blood pressure, wrinkles, arthritis, and hypothyroidism.

Menopause causes: Normal aging process. Metaphysically, it is the fear of no longer being wanted.

PMS symptoms:

Vata constitution: Lower backache, abdominal cramps, tiredness, and fatigue.

Remedy: Apply warm sesame oil on the painful areas and rest. Ginger, ajwain, and fennel teas are suggested for pain relief.

Pitta constitution: Irritability, sadness, anger, anxiousness, and indigestion.

Remedy: Chamomile tea, coriander-fennel-cumin tea, Aloe Vera juice, coconut water, and rose water.

Herbs: Shatavari, Purarnava, and Shankhapushpi.

Kapha constitution: Weight gain, water retention, and swelling of breasts.

Remedy: Ajwain, fenugreek, and cumin teas.

PMS causes: PMS is related to hormone changes that happen during the menstrual cycle and can be related to genetics.

Ayurvedic connotation: Menstrual issues and menopause can create imbalances in the three doshas due to lifestyle habits and intake of certain foods (e.g., processed foods).

Menstrual Symptoms and Menopause (Continued)

Suggested Remedies:

Diet:

Vata: Avocado, mustard greens, ghee, cooked leafy greens, nuts (pecans, walnuts, and almonds) and sesame seeds.

Pitta: Coconut, fennel, coriander, cumin, cardamom, saffron, avocado, asparagus, and sunflower seeds.

Kapha: Kale, bok choy, collard greens, mustard greens, green tea, and sesame seeds.

Lifestyle: Balanced lifestyle with regular daily routine (Dinacharya) and OM meditation every morning.

Yoga: Forward Bend, Chair, Warrior II, Hero, Cobbler, Bridge, Spinal Twist, and Corpse poses.

Pranayama: Shitali and Nadi-Shodhan.

Herbs:

Vata: Shatavari and Dashamoola.

Pitta: Aloe vera and Ashok.

Kapha: Aloe vera, Guggul, Dashamoola, and Ashok.

Migraines

Symptoms: A migraine is a common form of headache that is believed to occur as a result of complex interactions between the nervous system and the vascular system, as well as alterations in brain chemicals. It is an intense, pounding pain in the temple; the pain can be unilateral or bilateral, with nausea, diarrhea, facial pallor, cold hands and feet, and sensitivity to light and sound. A migraine can last between four and seventy-two hours.

Causes: Migraines may be caused by changes in the brainstem and its interactions with the trigeminal nerve, a major pain pathway. Imbalances in brain chemicals, including serotonin—which helps regulate pain in the nervous system—may also be involved. The causes could be genetics, hormonal changes in women, stress, foods (e.g., caffeine, alcohol, salty and processed foods), sensory stimuli, physical factors (intense physical exertion), and certain medications. Metaphysically, it is due to feeling driven, pressured, and fearful of letting someone in too close.

Ayurvedic connotation: Primarily a Pitta imbalance, it is an overreaction to any external stimuli or Pitta-provoking foods. Vata individuals have migraines that are more neurological in nature, causing strong headaches and vertigo, which can lead to cervical spondylitis. Generally, this is not associated with a Kapha constitution.

Suggested Remedies:

Diet: In general, items such as soups with ghee, ginger, fennel, and ajwain tea. It is best to avoid alcohol and red meat.

Vata: Freshly cooked root vegetables (squash, zucchini), soaked nuts (walnuts and almonds), soaked sesame seeds, poppy seeds, and more fluids (water) to hydrate. The recommendation is to eliminate acidic and processed foods, since they cause dehydration, accumulation of toxins, and inflammation.

Pitta: Aloe vera, buttermilk, almond milk; cooling teas made with cardamom, fenugreek, coriander, and mint. Consume dark raisins, almonds, and sunflower seeds.

Lifestyle: Reduce stress, sun exposure, and working long hours. It is suggested for Pitta individuals to swim in the early morning or evening.

Yoga: Forward-Bend, Half-Plow, Bridge, and Legs-Up-the-Wall poses.

Pranayama: Anuloma-Viloma, Kapalabhati, Shitkari, and Ujjayi.

Herbs:

Vata: Ginger, Cinnamon, Turmeric, Rasna, and Ashwagandha.

Pitta: Amalaki, Guduchi, Triphala, and Aloe Vera.

Obesity

Symptoms: It is when excess fat builds up in the adipose tissue and can be evident through an enlarged stomach, waist, thighs, or butt, resulting in fatigue.

Causes: One consumes more calories than are burned; it is also aggravated by genetics. Processed foods and foods high in sugar and fat contribute to rapid weight gain. Sedentary lifestyle and inactivity aggravates weight gain. Metaphysically it is due to fear, insecurity, and a deep need for emotional protection.

Ayurvedic connotation: This Kapha imbalance, due to excess intake of sugar, starch, fats, and decreased activity levels, can cause an imbalance in fat metabolism, resulting in deposits of excess adipose tissue.

Suggested Remedies:

Diet: Eating at the right time and in the correct proportions. Include leafy green vegetables, lentils, fish, chicken, and high-protein and nongluten grains such as quinoa, millet, and ragi.

Lifestyle: Increase physical activity / yoga and Pranayama for improving the metabolic fire.

Yoga: Raised Arm, Forward-Bend, Mountain, Cobra, Eagle, Upward Bow, Wind-Relieving, Cow, and Surya Namaskar poses.

Pranayama: Anuloma-Viloma, Kapalabhati, and Bhastrika.

Herbs: Triphala Guggul, Nedohar Guggul, Lasunadi, Punarnava, Dashamoola, and Ashwagandha.

Common Ailments and the Suggested Ayurvedic Remedies

Premature Gray Hair and Hair Loss

Symptoms: Graying of hair before the age of thirty-five, due to the reduction of melanin production in hair follicles. Hair shedding or hair thinning occurs between the ages of thirty and sixty.

Causes: Nutrition deficiency (of vitamin B, iron, copper and iodine), crash diets, stress, heredity, medical conditions (thyroid imbalance), childbirth, excessive heating of hair (high use of an electrical dryer), physical or emotional stress, hormonal changes, and an unclean scalp. Metaphysically, it is due to stress and feeling under pressure.

Ayurvedic connotation: It is a Pitta disorder due to excessive heat or chemicals applied to the hair.

Suggested Remedies:

Diet: Iron-rich, green leafy vegetables (spinach, kale, collard greens, and cilantro), calcium-rich foods such as dairy products, seeds (sesame), nuts (almonds), coconut, brown rice, fish, and coconut milk.

Lifestyle: Regular sleep patterns (avoid late nights), and avoid excessive spices, alcohol, caffeine, smoking, or any overly stimulating substances. A proper Dinacharya routine must be followed. Massage the scalp with coconut or olive oil. Meditation is essential, since it helps calm the mind and reduce stress.

Yoga: Fish, Half-Tortoise, Corpse, Wind-Relieving, Shoulder Stand, Downward Dog, Camel, and Headstand poses.

Pranayama: Anuloma-Viloma and Bhastrika.

Herbs: Amalaki, Triphala, and Bhringraj.

Rheumatoid Arthritis

Symptoms: It is an autoimmune disease where the body's immune system attacks normal joint tissues, causing inflammation of the joint lining. The symptoms include pain or stiffness in the morning lasting more than an hour; fatigue; inflammation in the wrists, fingers, neck, shoulders, feet, knees, and ankles; low bone density; dryness of the synovial fluid; and high blood pressure.

Causes: The cause is unknown but is potentially attributed to genetics or environmental factors. Metaphysically, it is due to a feeling of being victimized and a lack of love.

Ayurvedic connotation: A Vata imbalance due to blockages in the pathway by Ama. The blockages in certain parts of the body affect the related joints, but as the disease advances, the toxins get pushed to more areas in the body.

Suggested Remedies:

Diet: Toxin-reducing vegetarian diet including roasted and cooked grains such as quinoa, barley, millet, brown rice, and lentils; moong soup; green leafy vegetables; fruits; few root vegetables; nuts; and seeds. It is advised to avoid raw, cold, congestive food such as smoothies, juices, yogurt, cheese, and bread.

Lifestyle: Warm oil (sesame or medicated [*Mahanarayana*] oils) massage or hot compress massage with ginger and ajwain powder on the swollen joints. During the inactive phases of inflammation, gentle exercise (walking and stretching) and yoga is suggested. Swimming / aquatic exercises are beneficial.

Yoga: Easy Pose, Corpse, and Surya Namaskar poses.

Stretching: Neck Tilt and Turn, Wrist Bend, Shoulder Stretch, and Ankle Rotation exercises.

Pranayama: Kapalabhati.

Herbs: Guggul formulas. *(Please consult with an Ayurvedacharya for more information.)*

Sciatica

Symptoms: A pain that affects the sciatic nerve, extending from the lower back down to the back of each leg. The symptoms are pain, tingling or a burning sensation down the leg, numbness or difficulty moving the leg or foot, a pain on one side of the rear, and a shooting pain that makes standing up difficult.

Causes: Irritation of the root of the lumbar or lumbosacral spine, pregnancy, weight gain, lack of exercise, wearing high heels constantly, and sleeping on a soft mattress. Metaphysically, it is due to a lack of support or love, and a feeling of desperation.

Ayurvedic connotation: A Vata imbalance due to compression in the lumbar spine, pinching the sciatic nerve.

Suggested Remedies:

Diet: A healthful Vata-balancing diet with warm food is recommended.

Lifestyle: OM meditation, Ayurvedic treatments such as hot-stone massage, oil massages (sesame oil), *Kati-Basti* and *Pinda Sveda* therapies, regular exercise, and yoga (traction poses).

Yoga: Hand-to-Toe Forward-Bend, Extended Triangle, Downward-Facing Dog, and Half-Moon poses.

Pranayama: Anuloma-Viloma and Nadi-Shodhan.

Herbs: Rasna, Dashamoola, and Guggul formulas. *(Please consult with an Ayurvedacharya for more information.)*

Spondylitis

Symptoms: It is the inflammation of one or more vertebrae in the spine. The symptoms include back, leg, and hip pain; spinal deformity or curvature; abnormal nerve sensations in the back, thigh, and leg; bladder incontinence; decreased mobility due to pain; decreased muscle strength; and sexual dysfunction.

Causes: Osteoarthritis and rheumatoid arthritis, spinal injury or infection, and tuberculosis. Metaphysically, it is due to a rigid value system.

Ayurvedic connotation: It is a Vata imbalance that causes constriction, spasms in the muscles, and degenerative changes in the vertebrae discs, causing pain, stiffness, and lack of mobility.

Suggested Remedies:

Diet: Vata-reducing diet—plenty of fresh cooked vegetables, lentils, whole grains, warm milk, fruits (but avoid sour or acidic fruits such as grapefruit, pineapple), and root vegetables, using a good amount of ghee.

Lifestyle: OM meditation and warm oil massages (heat and lubrication) help reduce the symptoms and balance Vata.

Yoga: Cobra, Bridge, Plank, and Lotus poses.

Pranayama: Kapalabhati, Anuloma-Viloma, Bhastrika, Brahmari, Udgeeth, and Ujjayi.

Herbs: Dashamoola and Guggul formulas. *(Please consult an Ayurvedacharya for more information.)*

Stress

Symptoms: A feeling of being pressured, and that everything seems to be too much. The initial symptoms are anxiousness, nervousness, distraction, internal pressure, excessive worry, and changes in sleep patterns. The long-term symptoms include excessive fatigue, headaches, nausea, diarrhea, chest pain, dizziness, shortness of breath, hyperventilation, and thoughts of hurting oneself.

Causes: It can be caused by physical or emotional stimuli—work, relationship issues, social and financial problems, a lack of a support network, and medical illness. Metaphysically, it is due to feeling tired of life and stuck in a never-ending cycle that is not in keeping with inner peace.

Ayurvedic connotation: Stress is a lack of ability to handle the internal and external circumstances. One can display more Vata-related imbalances such as panic attacks, tremors, and anxiousness. Pitta-related stresses manifest as anger, heat flush, irritability, lack of interest in life, diarrhea, and even suicidal ideation. Kapha-related symptoms are inertia, depression, and overeating.

Suggested Remedies:

Diet: Eating fresh, natural, seasonal foods in a healthful and balanced diet. Include chamomile and valerian teas. Avoid caffeine and other stimulants, as well as synthetic sugars and preservatives.

Lifestyle: Sankalp meditation (meditation with intent), yoga, Pranayama, developing a creative hobby (group dancing or singing or sports), and getting involved in social activities.

Yoga: Child's Pose, Corpse, Bridge, Forward-Bend, Downward-Facing Dog, and Anjali Mudra poses.

Pranayama: Anuloma-Viloma, Ujjayi, Bhastrika, Kapalabhati, Brahmari, and Nadi-Shodhan.

Herbs: Brahmi, Ashwagandha, Shankhapushpi, and Jatamansi.

Temporomandibular Joint (TMJ) Issues

Symptoms: Problems with jaw, jaw joints, and the facial muscles controlling actions such as chewing

Causes: The cause is unknown, but some potential causes could be an injury to the jaw, grinding or clenching of the teeth, rheumatoid arthritis, stress that leads to tightening of facial muscles, and any dislocations. Metaphysically, it is anger, resentment, and not being able to let go.

Ayurvedic connotation: This is a Vata imbalance and a way to express psychological stress when the environmental conditions are difficult. Nervousness and anxiety are expressed through tightness in the TMJ and through symptoms such as grinding.

Suggested Remedies:

Diet: Warm, cooked, wholesome food with moisture and lubrication. Healthful fats such as ghee, soaked nuts, and avocado.

Lifestyle: Sesame oil in the ear or swishing oil in the mouth. The application of oil on the facial *marma points* is beneficial.

Shiro Basti—Massage oil on the head and leave it in for half an hour. Use medicated or coconut oil.

Shirodhara—Drip oil over the head and forehead, resulting in instant relaxation.

Yoga: Downward-Facing Dog, Upward-Facing Dog, Shoulder Stand, and Legs-Up-the-Wall poses (*Note:* Avoid Headstand Pose, since it can put more pressure on the TMJ).

Pranayama: Anuloma-Viloma.

Herbs: Brahmi, Ashwagandha, and Jatamansi.

Thyroid Issues

Symptoms: Due to overactivity of the thyroid gland, an excessive amount of thyroid hormones can be produced, resulting in hyperthyroidism. If there is underactivity of the gland, a deficiency of thyroid hormones results, causing hypothyroidism. The symptoms of hypothyroidism are fatigue, mental fogginess, constipation, dry skin, feeling cold, fluid retention, depression, and prolonged menstrual bleeding. The symptoms of hyperthyroidism are heat intolerance, excessive sweating, agitation, increased bowel movements, weight loss, fatigue, rapid heart rate, decreased concentration, and irregular menstrual flow.

Causes: Genetics, exposure to radiation, menopause, smoking, exposure to chemicals, and chronic fatigue syndrome. Metaphysically, it is due to feeling repressed and not being able to do what one desires.

Ayurvedic connotation:

Hypothyroidism: Imbalance in Kapha energy, which causes a lot of heaviness, weight gain, inertia, lack of appetite, depression, water retention, and overall slowing of metabolism.

Hyperthyroidism: It is a Vata imbalance, which causes anxiousness, nervousness, weight loss, nodular swelling in the thyroid, restlessness, insomnia, tremors, and hair loss.

Thyroid Issues (Continued)

Suggested Remedies:

Diet:

Hypothyroidism: Light roasted whole grains, fiber, lentils, and green leafy vegetables. Avoid toxin-increasing foods (congestive, processed, stale foods that cause heaviness), yogurt, cheese, and bread.

Hyperthyroidism: Vata-pacifying, nourishing, hydrating, lubricating foods (use ghee, soaked sesame, almonds, and walnuts), warm cooked foods, soups, broths, root vegetables, and seaweed. Avoid raw or processed foods.

Lifestyle:

Hypothyroidism: A daily routine of yoga and Pranayama, and additional exercises such as walking, swimming, or other group activities or sports.

Hyperthyroidism: Gentle exercises, yoga, and meditation along with calming and relaxing activities such as music or golf.

Yoga: Cat, Cobra, Bow, Fish, Boat, Head-to-Toe, Lotus, Wind-Relieving, Shoulder Stand, Lion, Camel, Tree, and Raised Foot poses.

Pranayama: Shitali, Sheethkari, Ujjayi, Bhastrika, and Surya Bhedhan.

Herbs:

Hypothyroidism: Ashwagandha, Dashamoola, Punarnava, and Triphala Guggul.

Hyperthyroidism: Kanchanar Guggul and Brahmi.

Chapter 22
Understanding of Herbs

(Please ensure that an Ayurvedic doctor or Ayurvedacharya is consulted for your specific ailments or needs before using any of the herbs described below.)

No.	Herb	Description
1.	Amalaki (Indian gooseberry)	Amalaki is high in antioxidants and vitamin C, facilitates digestive health, and aids with relieving constipation. It helps remove excess heat from the gastrointestinal tract and supports regular elimination. It is also known to support the functioning of the liver and heart and is good for healthy nails, hair, teeth, and bones.
2.	Ashok	It is known for menstrual-related problems, especially when there is excessive bleeding. Ashok has antibacterial properties. It is known to be healing for ailments such as uterine infections, rheumatoid arthritis, wounds, and neurological disorders.
3.	Ashwagandha	It has a carminative effect and relaxes the nervous system. It is used to reduce Vata-related disorders such as muscle pain, anxiety, and wrinkles in the skin. It is also known to reduce joint pains, lower cholesterol, and strengthen the immune system.
4.	Brahmi	This herb enhances memory and has been used to treat epilepsy, insomnia, depression, and schizophrenia. Brahmi is used as a memory booster, removes stress, and improves brain cell function. It improves the functioning of the liver, lungs, and kidneys and induces hair and nail growth. It can be used to treat Alzheimer's disease, Parkinson's disease, bronchitis, arthritis, and other inflammatory conditions.
5.	Bhringraj	This herb is used externally to address ailments such as athlete's foot, eczema, dermatitis, and hair loss. It is used to purify blood, resolve skin disorders, and enhance vision and hearing. The anti-inflammatory quality reduces pain and fever.

No.	Herb	Description
6.	Castor oil	This is a vegetable oil obtained from the seeds of the castor plant. It is commonly used as a laxative. It is known to help with headaches, inflammatory conditions, skin disorders, sinusitis, and muscle pains; it also enhances memory.
7.	Dashamoola	Dashamoola is a combination of ten herbs used to pacify Vata. It consists of herbs such as bilva root, agnimantha root, shyonaka root, patala root, kashmari root, bruhati root, kantakari root, shalaparni root, prushniparni root, and gokshura root. It is used to treat inflammatory conditions, fever, bronchitis, asthma, cough, flatulence, arthritis, sciatica, and other Vata-related disorders.
8.	Gotukola	This herb has antiviral, antibacterial, anti-inflammatory, and diuretic properties. It reduces anxiety and improves mental clarity. The herb is used to heal respiratory infection, hepatitis, fever, asthma, stomach ulcers, psoriasis, and varicose vein issues.
9.	Gudmar	It is used for hyperglycemia, obesity, high cholesterol, anemia, reduces blood sugar levels [controls sugar cravings], and aids in the treatment of constipation and jaundice *(Note: Please consult an Ayurvedacharya if you are pregnant or breast-feeding.)*
10.	Guduchi	Guduchi is helpful with ailments such as gout, jaundice, asthma, skin disorders, diarrhea, and diabetes. The herb helps control cholesterol and is usually prescribed for liver disorders. It is also used to manage postmenopausal symptoms such as nausea and fluid retention. It is known to balance all three doshas.
11.	Guggul	This herb has been used in Ayurveda for a long time as a weight-loss stimulant and to treat ailments such as urinary tract infection, hemorrhoids, acne, high cholesterol, and arthritis. *(Note: Please be advised that this may have side effects such as headaches and nausea. Please consult an Ayurvedacharya before use.)*
12.	Haritaki	It has digestive, anti-inflammatory properties and is also an aphrodisiac. It is known to fight constipation, cough, cold, and is also known to cure blindness. This herb removes excess Vata, cleanses the system, and rejuvenates the seven *Dhatus*.

Understanding of Herbs

No.	Herb	Description
13.	Jatamansi (spikenard)	Jatamansi is a memory enhancer and is an antispasmodic. It imparts calm and peace, reduces stress and anxiety, is an antidepressant, and increases the levels of serotonin. It helps reduce diabetes and high blood pressure and is used to treat eye disorders, liver problems, sleep disorders, mental disorders, hyperactivity, Alzheimer's disease, gastric disorders, vertigo, hepatitis, autism, typhoid, and epilepsy.
14.	Kathalai (aloe vera)	Aloe vera juice contains protein, calcium, magnesium, zinc, vitamin B_{12}, and essential fatty acids. This plant has therapeutic values—healing and rejuvenating qualities. It is used for skin treatments and to maintain a healthy digestive system, reduces the chafing of the nose, and helps heal wounds. The juice of this plant aids in weight loss and improves immunity. Aloe works on membranes, epithelial tissue (skin), lungs, and sinuses.
15.	Kutaj	Kutaj is useful in treating diarrhea, arthritis, colitis, malabsorption, ulcers, jaundice, and pulmonary problems. It also improves bowel movements and enhances the functioning of the digestive tract.
16.	Lasunadi	It is used in the treatment of diarrhea, anorexia, and other gastrointestinal tract–related diseases. It reduces gastric, colic pain, and arthritis pain. It treats liver disorders, asthma, and lung infections.
17.	Licorice	The licorice extract acts as a sweetener and is generally used in different kinds of candy. Licorice has an antiviral quality. It is used to heal stomach ailments, including ulcers, as well as diseases such as IBS and Crohn's disease. Licorice has also been beneficial in the treatment of autoimmune diseases such as lupus and rheumatoid arthritis.
18.	Manjistha	This is one of the best blood purifiers. Manjistha improves the functioning of the liver and can be used to prevent kidney stones and skin disorders. It has anti-inflammatory qualities.
19.	Neem	This is a blood cleanser that controls high blood sugar levels. Neem has antifungal, antidiabetic, antibacterial, and antiviral qualities. It is used for healthy hair, to improve the functioning of the liver, for blood detoxification, and in treating certain skin diseases. Neem oil is used in toothpastes, soaps, shampoos, and facial creams.

No.	Herb	Description
20.	Punarnava	This herb increases vigor and vitality in the body. It balances the digestive system and alleviates fluid retention, liver issues, respiratory problems, anemia, diabetes, asthma, abdominal pain, kidney failure, swelling in the joints, and high cholesterol.
21.	Rasna	This is used for any issues with the nervous system, sciatica, constipation, and flatulence. Rasna is also useful for asthma, bronchitis, chest pain, rheumatoid arthritis, and other Vata-related disorders.
22.	Sandalwood	Sandalwood is known for its antiseptic and disinfectant qualities. It is used to moisturize the skin and treat ailments such as eczema or psoriasis. It can diminish scars and blemishes on the skin. Sandalwood also has anti-inflammatory and antispasmodic properties used to treat high blood pressure, inflammation of the urinary system, viral infections, depression, spasms in the nerves and muscles, in addition to enhancing emotional well-being.
23.	Shankhapushpi	Shankhapushpi is known to stimulate the brain, promote the intellect, and improve memory, concentration, complexion, and appetite. It is known to treat insomnia, chronic constipation, abdominal pain, and mental and physical exhaustion.
24.	Shatavari	Shatavari is known for fertility benefits for men and women, is a hormone balancer, and aids with ovarian cysts and uterine fibroids. It has antioxidant, antibacterial, digestive, and adaptogenic properties, which can heal colitis, heartburn, and gastrointestinal infections.
25.	Trikatu	This is a mixture that equally contains the fruits of black pepper, Indian long pepper, and ginger. This herb supports digestion, respiration, and the digestive fire to aid in the breakdown of food and the absorption of nutrients. Trikatu is anti-inflammatory, rejuvenating the body cells by restoring normal blood flow to the cells.
26.	Triphala	This is a mild laxative that cleanses the gastrointestinal tract and is a blood cleanser. It is composed of three herbs—Amalaki, Haritaki, and vibhitaki. It is high in vitamin C and antioxidants.

Chapter 23
Ayurvedic and Tantric View on Sexual Healing

One of the interpretations of the beautiful carvings in the Khajuraho temples in India is that they are an expression of an experience of divine ecstacy. The Ayurvedic and Tantric texts have elucidated that the body is a *temple of God* and that sexual energy is a creative force—a pure energy that has been provided as a means for self-realization, rather than for just pleasure or procreation.

Ayurveda's perspective is that one must judiciously indulge in sexual activity. It begins with complete respect for one another in the partnership. Sexual union allows for the expansion of consciousness, opening your heart to love yourself and your partner on a spiritual level. It allows you to try to establish an unconditional love relationship between the "*I*" and the "*I AM*" or "*Paramatma*" (our higher self).

In practical terms, Ayurveda has advised us with the following guidelines:

- During the act of intimacy, it is suggested for one partner to lie on his or her left side; the one (male or female) who wants more nurturing should lie on the inside, enveloped by the other. Then both partners can rest their hands on the heart of the person lying inside, and breathe slowly and deeply. This will aid in promoting positive energy flow in the Chakras. Inhaling and exhaling together creates a stronger love connection and harmony.
- Another posture is to put a hand on each other's hearts while in a seated position in order to feel a higher, positive vibration. The Chakras and energy in the body are in constant flow, so by sending positive and loving thoughts toward one another, it is possible to create a higher vibration and a more harmonious reality between the two souls.
- Sex is meant to revitalize our entire system energetically right down to each cell. If it is done with consciousness, it opens our energy channels

to bring about a balance in the mind-body-spirit.
- There is male and female energy in both men and women, and the aim is to bring about a unification and balance of these two energies.
- Ayurveda expresses that you must understand yourself physically, emotionally, and spiritually for complete balance. Your body requires not only food to exist, but also an assimilation of your emotional, sensual, and sexual needs. It is best to use food as a balance to sensuality and sexuality rather than a substitute.
- An ideal partnership or marriage is when there exists a mutual respect in the partnership as spiritual beings. It is when a woman loves her husband or partner as a *guru* (shiva) and the husband or partner loves and respects her as a *goddess* (shakti). The two partners are spiritually equal; the man is not superior to the woman, and the act of sex or loving is a means to transform—to become greater than when they were alone.
- Unrestricted sexual activity is not propounded; it is detrimental to your health because it can cause a strain on the nerves and body tissues and can increase dryness or irritability in a person.
- Sex is not advised during illness, since it depletes *Ojas*.
- More sexual activity is suggested for winter rather than summer months.
- Sex should be avoided after a heavy meal or during pregnancy or menstruation.

Sexuality as a spiritual healing method was practiced more than five thousand years ago through the ancient spiritual practice of Tantra.

The esoteric teachings of Tantra have often been labeled as *secret* or *forbidden*. In recent times, there has been a rising integration between Western medicine and the Eastern tradition of mind-body consciousness for healing. Today, there is a deeper comprehension of Eastern thought, and quantum physicists are more accepting of the idea of energy flows in the material world, including our bodies.

The ancient yogic practice of Tantra propounded this notion of nonduality more than five thousand years ago. It emphasized that there was no separation between the external or material world and the spiritual world, especially in the human body, where sexuality is seen as a spiritual healing force. Tantra views the body as a manifestation of the spirit and sexual energy to be the life force of the Universe. It is by making the body pure and strong through asana, pranayama, meditation, mudras, and mantras that the body can become a vehicle for ending suffering, negative imbalances, and for attaining liberation.

The word *Tantra* comes from the combination of two Sanskrit words—*Tanoti* (expansion) and *Treyati* (liberation). In particular, it refers to the pathway from ignorance to enlightenment and literally means *continuum* or *the expansion of consciousness*. It is a method to expand the mind and liberate dormant potential energy. Tantra is about being fully in the present moment and engaging with yourself and your partner at the most intimate level. The orgasmic journey activates the nervous system and awakens the healing capabilities inside the body. This allows a complete energy flow in mind and body, aids in removing blockages, alleviates any pain (physical or emotional), and elevates the energy quotient in the body. It is about experiencing pleasure to the fullest along with being a means of spiritual healing. In Tantra, one learns to slow down, go within, completely surrender, and open one's entire being to receiving the highest energy in the present moment.

Please note: The above is not a suggestion to attempt Tantra on your own or be involved in any kind of irresponsible sexual activity just for pleasure or procreation. The explanation of Tantra above is meant to provide a basic understanding of an ancient Vedic spiritual healing method.

Chapter 24
Ongoing Maintenance as per Ayurveda

Nature has different seasons and colors. There are six seasons of two months each:
- The *Vata* season is fall/autumn (mid-September to mid-November). During Vata season, individuals move toward wanting warm temperatures/foods along with Vata-pacifying foods. It is suggested to avoid leftovers or canned foods, since they aggravate Vata. It is good to massage the body with basil or eucalyptus oil.
- The *Kapha* season is early through late winter (mid-November to mid-March). During the Kapha season, it is preferable to eat warm, stimulating food rather than cold or oily food. It is a time to focus on a more intense exercise routine and apply body masks using rosemary or fenugreek.
- The *Pitta* seasons are spring and summer (mid-March to mid-July). During Pitta season, you are advised to eat wholesome, cooling, and calming foods. It is suggested to avoid hot, spicy, or pungent foods. It is a time to enjoy nature and follow a water-based exercise routine, do yoga in the early mornings, and apply body masks using Neem, corn flour, and clay.

Ayurveda believes that the two main factors that affect good health are nutrition and modifications in lifestyle according to your specific constitution. The outcome is good physical, mental, and emotional health, along with a spiritual balance in keeping with the laws of nature.

There are some general rules or guidelines as per the science of Ayurveda:
- Exercising (walking, cardio exercises, or yoga) at least thirty minutes a day is necessary for good health.
- Ayurveda recommends at least ten minutes of meditation each morning

- and night. A calm mind leads to a sounder sleep at night.
- Food and lifestyle choices should be in accordance with your predominant dosha.
- Food should be fresh, usually cooked, tasty, and easy to digest.
- If you feel tired or heaviness in your stomach after a meal, it may be indicative of improper eating both in terms of quantity or quality.
- Avoid eating while watching television or while reading. Eat in peaceful and pleasant surroundings, in a silent, mindful manner, and avoid any emotional upsets while eating your food.
- Meals should be eaten at the same time each day.
- Lunch should be taken between 12 noon and 1:00 p.m., coinciding with the peak Pitta period, since Pitta is responsible for the digestive process.
- Sweet food turns sour in your digestive tract when the emotion present during the meal is negative. It is not advised to eat while you are upset—it is an insult to food, to the giver of foods, and to your body.
- You may sip warm water during the meal; avoid ice-cold water.
- It is advocated to have dinner between 6:00 p.m. and 7.00 p.m. Food should be light, cooked, and easy for digestion. Dinner should be eaten at least three hours before bedtime, since this interval allows the body ample time to digest the food.
- Sleeping on the left side will aid in digestion.

Guidelines for Maintenance—Vata Constitution:

- It is essential for Vata individuals to maintain a consistent daily routine.
- Avoid skipping meals and aim to eat in a peaceful environment while focusing on the actual process of eating.
- To promote circulation, do self-massage using sesame oil before you shower (*please do a self-test with the oil on a small area of your skin to ensure that there is no negative reaction/allergy/rash before applying all over your body*).
- Stay warm during the cold weather, using several layers of clothing.
- Walking is a beneficial exercise for Vata, especially in the morning for about twenty minutes.
- Vata individuals are encouraged to meditate for thirty minutes daily.
- Cooked foods, served hot or warm, are preferable for Vata constitution.

- Using some fat in the food—olive oil, coconut oil, or ghee—is advised.
- Include sweet, sour, and salty tastes in the food.
- Drink lots of warm water during the day.

Guidelines for Maintenance—Pitta Constitution:

- It is important for Pitta individuals to remain calm and cool physically and emotionally.
- Avoid coffee or tea on an empty stomach first thing in the morning.
- Avoid going out during the peak heat times of the day, especially if you are hungry.
- Avoid skipping meals or fasting. A sustaining lunch is essential for Pitta individuals.
- Use coconut oil for self-massage prior to the morning shower every day.
- Water-based exercises or activities are ideal for those with a Pitta constitution.
- Establish a balanced routine of work and rest.
- Meditation is beneficial for stress reduction.
- Sweet, bitter, and astringent tastes should be included in the food. Include ghee in the diet.
- Pomegranate juice is beneficial every morning.

Guidelines for Maintenance—Kapha Constitution:

- A proper exercise regime to maintain weight is advised, since Kapha tends to put on weight. Kapha constitution has strength and endurance, and this should be utilized through optimum activity or exercise to resist lethargy.
- Drinking hot water or bathing in hot water is proposed.
- Steam inhalations and steam baths or sauna sessions are good for Kapha. Body massage is beneficial.
- A diet with a focus on pungent, bitter, and astringent tastes is suggested.
- Foods that are cooked without much water or oil and those that are light, dry, and flavored with spices are preferable.
- Late-night snacking should be avoided.
- Pursuing new projects, activities, thoughts, and ideas keeps Kapha people stimulated and active.

Conclusion

It is said that real change comes from the inside out. It is my understanding that true change does not happen overnight, since it is a fundamental shift in thought and attitude, and, most importantly, an ability to explore into the unknown with the intrinsic belief that there is some greater lesson waiting to be grasped. It is this learning exercise that, in hindsight, brings more satisfaction than the outcome—especially if the journey of transformation is savored on a moment-to-moment basis.

> *Only in growth, reform, and change, paradoxically enough, is true security to be found.*[1]
>
> —Anne Morrow Lindbergh

This experience has been sublime for me personally, and I trust that this book has been beneficial for you too. I have fully enjoyed this creative experience by the grace of *Paramatma* and request to take your leave now. I am grateful to the *Universe* and *thank each one of you* for giving me the opportunity to be of service to you.

> *You are everything that is, your thoughts, your life, your dreams come true. You are everything you choose to be. You are as unlimited as the endless universe.*[2]
>
> —Shad Helmstetter

Namaste and love,
Vishnupriya.

Notes

Introduction
1. Helen Exley, ed., Wisdom for the New Millennium (Walford, UK: Exley, 1999).

Chapter 3
1. Asaido, Tel, "Charaka Samhita Bio," EdibleWildFood, 2020, https://www.ediblewildfood.com/bios/charaka-samhita.aspx.

Chapter 4
1. "Height and Weight Charts," Health Check Systems, n.d., https://www.healthchecksystems.com/heightweightchart.htm.
2. Ibid.

Chapter 21
1. "Disease," Lexico Dictionaries, https://www.lexico.com/en/definition/disease.

Conclusion
1. Helen Exley, ed., Wisdom for the New Millennium (Walford, UK: Exley, 1999).
2. Ibid.

Glossary

Abhayanga-dosha: Specific herbal oil massage to loosen toxins from the tissues

Adho Mukha Svanasana / Downward-Facing Dog: Yoga Asana or posture

Agni: Digestive fire, responsible for all digestive and metabolic processes in the body

air: One of the natural elements and part of the Panchamahabhutas

Ajna: Sixth primary Chakra, or third-eye Chakra

Ama: Buildup of toxins in the body

Amalaki: *Phyllanthus emblica* or Indian gooseberry

Anhata: Fourth primary Chakra, or heart Chakra

Anjali: The quantity that fits the two cupped palms held close together

anti-inflammatory: Product or substance that reduces inflammation or swelling

antiseptic: Product or substance that cleanses and prevents the development of organisms

Anuloma-Viloma: Pranayama or breathing technique, specifically alternate nostril breathing

aphrodisiac: Sexual stimulant that increases vitality and builds organs

Artha: One of the principal aims of life, specifically wealth

Asana: Yoga posture

Ashok: *Saraca asoca*—an Ayurvedic herb used in healing bleeding disorders related to a gynecological condition

astringent: One of the six tastes or Rasa in Ayurveda

asafoetida: Hing or spice that is used to relieve stomach gas

Ashwagandha: *Withania somnifera* or Ayurvedic herb used to increase energy and reduce stress

Atharva Veda: The fourth Vedic text

Atma: Inner self or true self of an individual or soul

Ayu: Means life
Ayurveda: Five-thousand-year-old science of medicine and life from India
Ayurvedacharya: Ayurvedic doctor
Balasana: Child's pose in yoga
Basti: Medicated enema
Bhastrika: Bellow's breath technique or Pranayama
Bhringraj: Ayurvedic herb that is a liver cleanser
Bhujangasana: Cobra pose in yoga
bitter: One of the six tastes or Rasa in Ayurveda
black pepper: A commonly used spice that is high in antioxidants
Brahmari: Bee-humming breathing technique or Pranayama
Brahmi: *Bacopa monnieri* or Ayurvedic herb that sharpens the brain and improves memory
cardamom: Green cardamom, which is a spice used in Ayurvedic cooking, or elettaria cardamomom, which is a digestive aid and breath freshener
carminative: Relieves intestinal gas, pain, bloating, and distention
Chakras: Energy vortexes in the body
Charaka: One of the principal contributors to Ayurveda and the compiler of the *Charaka Samhita*
Charaka Samhita: Sanskrit text on Ayurveda
cinnamon: Cinnamomum, or spice that is high in antioxidants, is anti-inflammatory, and lowers blood sugar levels
clove: Spice that is high in antioxidants and can improve liver health
consciousness: Awareness or perception or becoming awake
constitution: Qualities (physical, emotional, psychological) that are unique for each individual
coriander: Chinese parsley, a spice that has antioxidants and may promote gut health
cumin: A spice that promotes digestion and improves blood cholesterol
curry leaf: Native herb or spice of India that is high in antioxidants
Dashamoola: Ayurvedic herb that is used for pain and inflammatory disorders
Dhanurasana: Bow pose in yoga
Dharma: One of the four principal aims of life, specifically duty
Dhatus: Tissues in the body

Glossary

Dinacharya: Daily routine as described in Ayurveda

diuretic: Increases flushing out of liquids from the body, or urination

doshas: Biological energies found in the human body and mind

earth: One of the natural elements and part of the Panchamahabhutas

ether: One of the natural elements and part of the Panchamahabhutas

fenugreek: Spice that is good for reducing high cholesterol and high blood sugar

five senses: Sight, smell, sound, taste, touch

garlic: A plant of the onion family; helps with the common cold, improves cholesterol levels, and reduces blood pressure

ghee: Clarified butter

ginger: Spice that is anti-inflammatory and has an antioxidant effect

Gotukola: Ayurvedic herb for longevity

Gudmar: Ayurvedic herb that helps with diabetes and suppresses that craving for sweets or sugar

Guduchi: Ayurvedic herb that helps with infections, fever, and digestive disorders

Guggul: Ayurvedic herb that lowers cholesterol and triglycerides

Gunas: Quality or virtue

Halasana: Plow pose in yoga

Haritaki: Ayurvedic herb that is high in vitamin C, has an antioxidant effect, and is anti-inflammatory

healing: The process of becoming healthy again

holistic: Whole, treating mind-body-spirit

I AM: Higher consciousness, God

jaggery: Unrefined sugar product

Jatamansi: Ayurvedic herb that helps maintain a healthy nervous system and brain function (should be avoided during pregnancy)

Kama: One of the principal aims of life, specifically desire or love

Kanchanar Guggul: Ayurvedic herb for thyroid balancing

Kapalbhati: Skull-shining breathing technique or Pranayama

Kapha: dosha consisting of the elements of earth and water

Kathalai: Aloe vera

Kati-Basti: Ayurvedic healing treatment for lower back pain

Kundalini: Divine feminine energy located at the base of the spine

Kutaj: Ayurvedic herb for digestive issues and inflammation
Lasunadi: Ayurvedic herb for stomach problems and indigestion
licorice: Herb for gastrointestinal and respiratory issues
longevity of life: Long life
Malas: Waste products in the body
Manda: Slow
Manipura: Third primary Chakra, or solar plexus Chakra
Manjistha: Ayurvedic herb that fights inflammation and improves immunity
Mantra: Sacred sound or chant
Marjariasana: Cat and Cow pose in yoga
masala Dabba: Spice box
meditation: Practice of awareness or mindfulness to calm the mind
mindfulness: Attention to the now or present moment without judgment
Moksha: Salvation
Mooldhara: First primary Chakra, or root Chakra
Mudras: Symbolic gestures
mustard seed: Spice that contains selenium and has high anti-inflammatory effects
Nadi-Shodhan: Alternate-nostril breathing technique or Pranayama
Nasya: Nasal oil technique to soothe the nasal passages and reduce stress
Navasana: Boat pose in yoga
Neem: Indian lilac and Ayurvedic herb used for stomach ulcers, skin disease, and to prevent plaque in the mouth
nutmeg: Spice that is used for detoxification, indigestion, and increasing immunity
Ojas: Immunity
OM: Sacred sound, essence of consciousness or Atma
Panchamahabhutas: The five elements in nature; namely, earth, fire, air, space, and water
Panchakarma: Ayurvedic therapies for detoxification, cleansing, and rejuvenation
Paramatma: Absolute Atma, higher consciousness, God
Pavanmuktasana: Wind Release pose in yoga
Pinda Sveda: Ayurvedic massage and sweat therapy

Pitta: dosha consisting of the elements of fire and water
Prana: Life force
Prakruti: Unique individual constitution in Ayurveda
Pranayama: Breath control or technique
pungent: One of the six tastes or Rasa in Ayurveda
Punarnava: Ayurvedic herb is anti-inflammatory and has expectorant properties. It is used to remove excess fluid and rejuvenates the body.
Raktamoshana: Ayurvedic detoxification process, specifically blood-letting or blood detoxification
Rajasic: Guna that increases energy in the body (e.g., passion or action)
Rasa: Taste
Rasayana: Rejuvenation therapy in Ayurveda that restores the vitality of the body
red chili: A hot spice that is packed with vitamin C and antioxidants that support the immune system in the body
saffron: Expensive, fragrant spice that is a powerful antioxidant, treats depression, and is an aphrodisiac
Sahasrara: Seventh primary Chakra, or crown Chakra
Salamba Bhujangasana: Backward Bend or Sphinx pose in yoga
salty: One of the six tastes or Rasa in Ayurveda
Samyoga: Linking together or combination
sandalwood: Expensive spice that helps with depression and anxiety, is an aphrodisiac, and is used in religious ceremonies
Sankalp: Will or determination
Saptadhatu: The seven types of tissues in the body, including Rasa (fluids), rakta (blood), mamsa (muscle), medha (adipose), asthi (bone), majja (bone marrow), and shukra (hormones)
Sarvasana: Corpse pose in yoga
Sattvic: Guna that balances energy in the body (e.g., calm)
Seethkari: Hissing breath technique or Pranayama
space: One of the natural elements and part of the Panchamahabhutas
self-realization: Understanding and fulfilling one's true potential
Setu Bandha Sarvangasana: Bridge pose in yoga
sexuality: One's sexual preference or orientation
Shakti: Hindu goddess, divine cosmic feminine energy

Shankhapushpi: Ayurvedic herb that enhances concentration and relieves depression and fatigue,

Shatavari: Ayurvedic herb that increases vitality

Shiro Basti: Ayurvedic therapy of putting infused oil on the head; helps with mental illnesses

Shirodhara: Ayurvedic therapy using focused stream of herbal oils over the forehead to reduce stress and nervous tension

Shitali: Cooling breathing technique or Pranayama

Shiva: Adiyogi, is nothingness and the embodiment of power

sour: One of the six tastes or Rasa in Ayurveda

spice: Mix of herbs

spiritual healing: Balancing our spiritual body or soul

Supta Matsyendrasana: Spinal Twist pose in yoga

Surya Bhedhan: Single-nostril breathing technique or Pranayama

Surya Namaskar: Sun Salutation flow in yoga

Sushumna: Energy channel in the spinal cord

Susruta: Vedic physician in ancient times, author of the *Sushruta Samhita*

Sutrasthana: Knowledge of the medical aspects of Ayurveda in the *Sushruta Samhita*

Swadisthana: Second primary Chakra, or sacral Chakra

Swedana: Ayurvedic steam therapy

sweet: One of the six tastes or Rasa in Ayurveda

Tamasic: Guna that is negative energy in the body (e.g., lethargy, pessimism)

Tanoti: To extend, expand

Tantra: An ancient, Vedic spiritual system that enhances one's awareness to everything. It is exploring the feminine aspects of men and the masculine aspects of women (i.e., the Shiva-Shakti energy) to balance and grow spiritually. It is the weaving of energy expansion or union.

Tejas: Metabolic strength

Tiksha: Sharp and fiery Agni

transformation: Change or metamorphosis

Treyati: Liberation

Tridoshas: Three fundamental energies that govern our physical and emotional bodies

Trikatu: Ayurvedic herb that supports normal circulation and gastric functions

Trikonasana: Triangle pose in yoga

Triphala: Ayurvedic herb that acts as a laxative and helps with weight loss

turmeric: Contains curcumin; anti-inflammatory and used for pain, depression, high cholesterol, skin problems, and liver issues

Udgeeth: Chanting breath technique or Pranayama

Ujjayi: Victorious breath technique or Pranayama

Urdhva Mukha Svanasana: Upward-Facing Dog pose in yoga

Ustrasana: Camel pose in yoga

Uttanasana: Forward Bend pose in yoga

Vata: dosha consisting of the elements of air and space

Vedas: Ancient Hindu script: *Rig Veda*, *Yajur Veda*, *Atharva Veda*, and *Sama Veda*

Vikruti: dosha imbalance

Vipaka: Postdigestion effect

Virasana: Hero pose in yoga

Virechna: Purgative

Virya: Potency

Vishamagni: Irregular digestion

Vishuddha: Fifth primary Chakra, or throat Chakra

well-being: The state of being happy, comfortable, balanced, and positive

yoga: Union; to yoke, concentrate, practice to tone the physical body, calm the mind, and stay in the present moment for spiritual growth

Bibliography

Asaido, Tel. "Charaka Samhita Bio." EdibleWildFood, 2020. https://www.ediblewildfood.com/bios/charaka-samhita.aspx.

"Disease." Lexico Dictionaries. https://www.lexico.com/en/definition/disease.

Exley, Helen, ed. *Wisdom for the New Millennium*. Walford, UK: Exley, 1999.

"Height and Weight Charts." Health Check Systems, n.d. https://www.healthchecksystems.com/heightweightchart.htm.

Index

A
Abhayanga, 82
Adho Mukha Svanasana, 94
Agni, 4–5, 13, 20–21, 27, 53, 94, 102
air, 12, 14, 23, 29
Ajna, 92
Ama, 13, 20, 27, 80, 82, 95, 102, 116
Amalaki, 101, 103–104, 113, 115, 123, 126
anesthetic, 43
Anhata, 92
Anjali, 45, 119
antiseptic, 41–43, 126
Anuloma-Viloma, 96–102, 106, 108–109, 113–115, 117–120
aphrodisiac, 43, 124
Artha, 12
Asana, 129
Asanas, 129
Ashok, 112, 123
astringent, 24–26, 29–40, 108, 132
asafoetida, 39, 42, 52, 57, 60, 81, 106
Ashwagandha, 99, 113–114, 119–120, 122–123
Atharva Veda, 11
Atma, 88, 91
Ayu, 11
Ayurveda, 4–5, 7–8, 11–14, 20, 23–24, 27–28, 41, 45, 53, 80, 85–86, 95, 107, 124, 127–128, 130–131
Ayurvedacharya, 6–7, 41–42, 53, 77, 80, 82–83, 95, 98, 101, 103, 116–118, 123–124

B
Balasana, 94
Basti, 82–83, 117, 120
Bhastrika, 104, 108, 110, 114–115, 118–119, 122
Bhringraj, 115, 123
Bhujangasana, 94
bitter, 24–25, 29–35, 37–40, 47, 101, 132
black pepper, 39, 41–42, 52, 54, 56, 61–62, 64, 97, 108, 126
Brahmari, 99, 108–110, 118–119
Brahmi, 103–105, 110, 119–120, 122–123

C
cardamom, 39, 43, 52, 55–56, 73, 75, 77, 108–109, 112–113
carminative, 42–43, 123
chakra, 5, 91–93, 103

Index

chakras, 91, 93, 127
Charaka, 11
Charaka Samhita, 11
cinnamon, 39, 43, 52, 55, 76–77, 97, 101, 113
clove, 43, 55
consciousness, 9, 11, 14, 20, 28, 86, 127–129
constitution, 4, 7–8, 12–13, 15–16, 18–19, 21, 24, 29–40, 53, 77, 95, 103, 111, 113, 130–132,
coriander, 39, 42, 52, 60–61, 67–68, 70, 96, 104, 107–108, 111–113
cumin, 39, 42, 52, 55–56, 58–61, 67–70, 79, 81, 96, 99–101, 106–109, 111–112
curry leaf, 44, 71

D

Dashamoola, 106, 108–109, 112, 114, 117–118, 122, 124
Dhanurasana, 94
Dharma, 12
Dhatus, 124
Dinacharya, 99, 104, 112, 115
diuretic, 41–42, 124
dosha, 4, 7, 12, 14–15, 18–19, 24–25, 77, 85, 88, 95, 131
doshas, 12–15, 20, 23–25, 29, 54–76, 88, 111, 124

E

earth, 12, 14–15, 29
ether, 14

F

fenugreek, 39, 43, 46, 52, 57, 77–79, 101, 106–107, 109, 111, 113, 130
five senses, 10, 24, 95

G

garlic, 9, 25, 40, 44, 52, 55, 62, 78, 98, 107, 110
ghee, 36, 49, 51, 54, 57–60, 65, 67–69, 71, 73, 75, 80–81, 98, 104–105, 110, 112–113, 118, 120, 122, 132
ginger, 25, 40, 43, 52, 55, 57, 60–61, 63–64, 66–68, 70–71, 77, 81, 97–98, 100, 104, 107, 111, 113, 116, 126
Gotukola, 110, 124
Gudmar, 101, 124
Guduchi, 103, 113, 124
Guggul, 98, 101, 108–109, 112, 114, 116–118, 122, 124
Gunas, 14, 27

H

Halasana, 94
Haritaki, 100, 124, 126
healing, 5–7, 11–12, 20, 28, 41, 95, 123–125, 127–129
holistic, 11, 103

I

I AM, 6, 86–88, 127, 133

Index

J
jaggery, 37, 50, 73, 75, 106
Jatamansi, 119–120, 125

K
Kama, 12
Kanchanar Guggul, 122
Kapalbhati, 88, 96, 98
Kapha, 12–13, 15–19, 21, 24–25, 29–40, 53–54, 60–62, 65, 67–70, 72, 74, 79, 86, 88, 97, 108–109, 111–114, 119, 121, 130, 132
Kathalai, 125
Kati-Basti, 117
Kutaj, 107, 125

L
Lasunadi, 114, 125
licorice, 97, 99, 125
longevity of life, 11

M
Malas, 13, 20
Manda, 21
Manipura, 92
Manjistha, 102, 125
mantras, 110
Marjariasana, 94
masala Dabba, 41
meditation, 13, 20, 26, 80, 83, 86–89, 102–103, 105–107, 110, 112, 115, 117–119, 122, 129, 131–132
metabolism, 13, 15–16, 24, 41–42, 44, 98, 108, 114, 121

mindfulness, 5, 89–90
Moksha, 12
Mooldhara, 91
Mudras, 129
mustard seeds, 40, 44, 52, 56–57, 65, 67–68, 70

N
Nadi-Shodhan, 87, 102–103, 107–108, 112, 117, 119
Nasya, 82–83
natural, 8, 12, 23, 25, 29, 41–44, 82, 85, 90, 100, 102, 111, 119
Navasana, 94
Neem, 96, 102, 125, 130
nutmeg, 40, 44, 52, 64, 107

O
Ojas, 20–21, 28, 82, 128
OM, 107, 110, 112, 117–118
optimum health, 11, 20

P
Panchamahabhutas, 12
Panchakarma, 5, 21, 82–83
Paramatma, 6, 88, 91, 127, 133
Pavanmuktasana, 94
Pinda Sveda, 117
Pitta, 12–13, 15–19, 21, 23, 25, 29–40, 42, 53, 57, 61–63, 65, 68, 73, 76, 78, 85–86, 88, 96, 99, 101–103, 106, 108, 111–113, 115, 119, 130–132
Prana, 12, 21, 85, 87

Prakruti, 4, 12, 14–16
Pranayama, 5, 20, 26, 80, 83–84, 86–89, 96–110, 112–120, 122, 129
pungent, 24–26, 29–35, 37–40, 130, 132
Punarnava, 108–109, 114, 122, 126

R
Raktamoshana, 82
rajas, 14
Rajasic, 8–9, 27
Rasa, 4, 24, 29–40
Rasayana, 21, 139, 145
red chili, 40, 42, 52, 62–63, 67–68, 74
rejuvenation, 21, 83

S
saffron, 40, 43, 52, 54, 56, 77, 112
Sahasrara, 93
Salamba Bhujangasana, 94
salty, 9, 24–26, 31, 33, 36, 38–40, 113, 132
Samyoga, 11
sandalwood, 103, 108–109, 126
Sankalp, 119
Saptadhatu, 13
Sarvasana, 94
Sattva, 14
Sattvic, 8, 27–28
Seethkari, 103
space, 12, 14, 29
self-acceptance, 86
self-love, 9, 92, 96, 103
self-realization, 127

sensual living, 7
Setu Bandha Sarvangasana, 94
sexuality, 128
Shakti, 128
Shankhapushpi, 110–111, 119, 126
Shatavari, 106, 111–112
Shiro Basti, 120
Shirodhara, 83, 120
Shitali, 88, 96, 99, 103, 112, 122
Shiva, 128
sour, 24–26, 31–33, 36–37, 40, 50, 118, 131–132
spice, 41–44, 60
spiritual, 6–7, 11–12, 17, 28, 83, 87, 89, 91–93, 103, 127–130
spiritual healing, 6–7, 128–129
Supta Matsyendrasana, 94
surrender, 129
Surya Bhedhan, 122
Surya Namaskar, 94, 98, 102–103, 107, 114, 116
Sushumna, 91
Susruta, 11
Sutrasthana, 11
swadhisthana, 91
Swedana, 83
sweet, 16, 24–26, 29–40, 45, 47, 73, 77, 93, 96, 101, 131–132

T
tamas, 14
Tamasic, 8–9, 27
Tanoti, 129
Tantra, 128–129

taste, 10, 24–25, 29–41, 43, 54–57, 61–64, 66–70, 81, 89
Tejas, 21
Tiksha, 21
toxins, 13, 20–22, 27, 41, 44, 80, 82–83, 85, 102, 113, 116
transformation, 1, 7, 9, 14–15, 20, 133
Treyati, 129
Tridoshas, 42–43
Trikatu, 97, 99, 126
Trikonasana, 94
Triphala, 96, 100, 102, 108–109, 113–115, 122, 126
turmeric, 40–41, 52, 55–58, 60–61, 63, 65, 69–70, 81, 97, 101–103, 108, 113

U
Udgeeth, 118
Ujjayi, 99, 105, 113, 118–119, 122
Universe, 6, 12–14, 20, 85–88, 91–92, 129, 133
Urdhva Mukha Svanasana, 94
Ustrasana, 94
Uttanasana, 94

V
Vata, 12–19, 21, 23, 25, 29–40, 53–54, 56–57, 60–61, 63, 67, 72–73, 75–77, 85, 88, 97, 100, 105–106, 109–113, 116–124, 126, 130–132
Vedas, 11
Vikruti, 12
Vipaka, 24
Virasana, 94
Virechana, 82
Virya, 24
Vishamagni, 21
Vishuddha, 92

W
water, 12, 14–15, 22–23, 29, 33, 42, 44–45, 54–56, 58–63, 65, 69–71, 73–75, 78, 80–81, 86, 96, 98–100, 108–109, 111, 113, 121, 130–132
well-being, 7–8, 11–12, 22, 82, 84, 90, 126

Y
yoga, 5, 13, 80, 85–87, 94, 96–110, 112–120, 122, 130

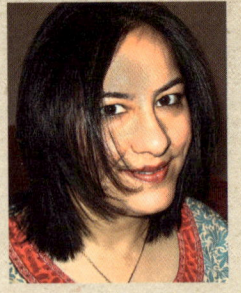

Vishnupriya Thacker is a certified holistic Ayurvedic wellness coach with a focus on mind-body-spirit well-being. She completed her training at the Institute of Integrative Integration with a focus on the science of Ayurveda, with guidance from an established Ayurvedic physician, Dr. Bapat, who in turn became the medical advisor for *Vedic Transformation*. Her knowledge in spiritual healing was obtained through exploring various spiritual/energy healing modalities such as Vedic spiritual guidance, reiki, chakra healing, crystal therapy, and violet flame healing. She is the founder and CEO of Vedic Synergy, an Ayurvedic wellness and spiritual-healing coaching practice in New York City. Their program offering "Rise like a Phoenix" has successfully empowered men and women to bring about a complete mind-body-soul transformation. Please visit www.vedicsynergy.com for more details. Namaste.